ENHANCING
FLEXIBILITY
&
MOBILITY

At-Home Exercises for Seniors

Table of Content

Chapter 1

Introduction to Flexibility and

Mobility for Seniors

Aging is inevitable and one of the most important stages of the human lifecycle. As humans age, they tend to undergo physical and physiological changes, significantly shaping their overall health and quality of life. One of the notable of these changes is the decline in their flexibility and mobility. So, as you are growing old, it is important to understand how flexibility and mobility play a part in improving and promoting your health, independence, and overall quality of life.

This is one of the biggest factors that motivated me and made me write this book. The main objective is to make you understand how flexibility and mobility can greatly help you improve your overall health and make you grow into a better person physically and physiologically as a senior. You might have been wondering what the connection between flexibility and mobility may be and how it can help you to improve your quality of life. You are in the right place, as I am ready to show you everything you need to know. Now, let's dive right into it.

How does aging affect flexibility and mobility in seniors?

Aging comes with a lot of physical and physiological changes that have a profound impact on an individual's flexibility and mobility. These changes are usually due to a combination of different intrinsic factors like genetics and extrinsic factors such as lifestyle choice and environmental factors. Understanding which one of the factors is responsible for your decline in flexibility will really aid in deciding the action that needs to be taken to better understand and improve your physiological health through close examination and proper management. Let's look at some of the ways in which aging can impede your flexibility and mobility as an adult.

1. Muscle Mass and Strength: one of the main factors that impact flexibility and mobility in seniors is the decrease in muscle mass and strength. This is an age-related condition known as sarcopenia. This process of sarcopenia usually begins at the early stage of adulthood, specifically at the approximate age of 30, but its acceleration usually becomes more pronounced at 50. The decline in muscle mass simply means a decrease in the amount of muscle available for an individual to support or move their body. This usually results in a reduction in human's overall strength and physical performance.

This prolonged loss of muscle and physical strength is usually partly due to hormonal change, specifically a decline in the decline in growth hormones and sex hormones like testosterone and estrogen. Moreover, decreasing your physical activities and insufficient protein intake can contribute to the development of sarcopenia and may also make it more noticeable and severe.

Sarcopenia tends to have a lot of implications that touch on several aspects of a senior's life. Some of the implications of this age-related condition on an individual include reduced muscle mass, decline in muscle strength, impaired physical performance, and increased vulnerability to injuries.

2. Connective Tissue Changes: The connective tissue changes, such as tendon and ligament elasticity, play a significant impact on a senior's flexibility and mobility. The connective tissues are responsible for stabilizing joints and supporting an individual's muscles, and aging can result in a decline in the elasticity of these tissues. This decline or loss of elasticity can make it difficult for these tissues to contract and expand effectively, limiting the range of motion in their joint. This will lead to a stiffened joint, making it difficult for seniors to perform some simple activities, resulting in discomfort and difficulty carrying out daily activities.

Moreover, the decline in flexibility in these connective tissues greatly impacts muscle function, which can affect muscle contraction efficiency. This will result in declined strength and power, affecting overall physical performance. Seniors with less pliable tendons and ligaments are at a higher risk of injuries such as sprains and strains during physical activity, leading to pain, reduced mobility, and extended recovery periods. These connective tissue changes can also exacerbate the symptoms of chronic conditions, making it particularly challenging to engage in exercises or physical therapy necessary for their management.

3. Joint Health: This is another factor that affects an individual's flexibility and mobility in seniors, as aging takes a toll on their joint health. Specifically, osteoarthritis is a condition common among aged people and greatly impacts an individual's joint well-being. This degenerative joint problem is known as "wear and tear" arthritis. It is usually caused by a gradual breakdown in cartilage, the protective tissue that cushions the end of the joint bone.

Osteoarthritis frequently causes symptoms such as joint pain, stiffness, and decreased range of motion. Affected joints may become inflamed, and pain may be felt during or after physical exercise. These symptoms can be especially difficult for seniors since they might interfere with everyday activities and diminish their quality of life.

Osteoarthritis can significantly affect a senior's flexibility and mobility. It is difficult for people to retain their independence, engage in regular physical activity, and carry out daily duties because of their stiffness, discomfort, and restricted range of motion. A more sedentary lifestyle may result from a mobility restriction over time, aggravating the problem and lowering overall joint health.

4. Balance and Coordination: As people age, their balance and coordination noticeably decline, significantly affecting their physical wellness. The decline in muscle strength, vision changes, and alterations in sensory perception all compromise these processes. Poor balance and coordination broadly influence day-to-day activities, making them more arduous and hazardous for elderly persons. Merely attempting to stay on one leg or traverse uneven terrain can amplify the danger of slips and resulting traumas.

Decreased balance and coordination can have a severe impact on seniors. The main worry is the heightened danger of falls that can produce harm, injuries, fractures, and declining trust in their movement abilities. These constrictions in balance and coordination can also lead to a decline in independence as seniors may require help with undertakings they could formerly achieve effortlessly. Moreover, the fear of falling can deter seniors from participating in physical and social activities, leading to social isolation, and negatively impacting their mental and emotional health.

5. Chronic Health Condition: Elderly individuals often face a heightened risk of developing chronic medical issues like diabetes and osteoporosis, which can greatly impede their flexibility and mobility. As people age, these types of illnesses become increasingly common, having a profound influence on bodily health, and ultimately impacting the general welfare of seniors.

Knowing how aging can affect your flexibility and mobility as a senior will help you understand if the decline in your flexibility and mobility results from aging. It will also let you know which challenges you are facing, create a better strategy to overcome them and enhance your flexibility and mobility even as you age.

It is important to note that these changes are usually irresistible due to aging. You must face it with an increase in age and body development. However, enhancing your physical and physiological health through regular exercise, proper nutrition, and lifestyle choices is still possible, which can help you improve your flexibility and mobility.

The Role of Flexibility in Maintaining Independence

Flexibility is a crucial component of physical well-being for older people and is critical in preserving their independence. The ability to complete day-to-day tasks and everyday movements without guidance directly correlates to flexibility. To further understand the need for flexibility in seniors, we must explore how it affects their independence and why individuals need to take it seriously to help maintain their independence and live a better life.

Imagine rousing one morning and discovering it nearly unimaginable to stoop down to fasten your laces or stretch out for that highly valued book perched on an elevated shelf. These are the routines we regularly ignore. However, they're strongly bound to senior's independence, and flexibility is important in making them achievable. The ability to move and expand comfortably permits seniors to perform these tasks independently.

Yet, flexibility does more than merely foster these routine tasks; it safeguards against sustaining wounds. Picture grasping a pot off the top compartment of a kitchen cupboard. With sound flexibility, this becomes a smooth, easy reach. Deficient in it, you might overstretch, resulting in a pulled muscle or, worse still, a fall. Those of advanced age with suppleness in their corner are less likely to experience strains, sprains, and additional painful injuries.

But attaining tall shelves and crouching down is not the only thing; flexibility is the answer to mobility. It is the difference between effortlessly rising from and settling into a chair or painfully enduring each movement. Mobility means you can roam your house and area without having a second thought, permitting you the freedom to explore and relish life's journeys independently.

Now, let's discuss joint health. A regular program of flexibility exercises, like moderate stretching, is beneficial to keeping articulations elastic and supple. This is profoundly important for individuals struggling with conditions like arthritis, which can harden joints and generate pain. It is possible to reduce some of that discomfort by upholding flexibility, a necessary component of maintaining independence.

There exists a psychological element to this matter as well. Enabling seniors to perform tasks on their own commonly leads to improved self-esteem. It is not merely concerned with finishing the task; it is associated with feeling competent and self-reliant, which can have a formidable effect on psychological welfare.

To cap off, let's consider the fall prevention. Falls are a substantial problem for older people, and flexibility can be a safeguard. Just think of that quick, surprising trip – your flexibility allows you to act fast and restore your stability. Seniors with better flexibility are more agile, and this agility is a key element in diminishing the chance of falls.

Thus, being flexible isn't just about lengthening one's muscles; it also involves expanding the possibilities of what elderly individuals can do autonomously, guarding their liberty, security, and health in general.

The Connection Between Mobility and Quality of Life

The relationship between mobility and the quality of life for seniors is unequivocally clear. Mobility, encompassing the capacity to move or ascend effortlessly and comfortably, whether it be striding, clambering upstairs, or just hauling oneself out of a chair, is highly necessary for the well-being of older individuals. Let us examine this association further to gain a more intensive appreciation.

Attending social functions and partaking in leisure activities can be much more gratifying when you have the mobility to do so. Without the ability to travel, you may miss out on the chance to visit family and friends or partake in the community events that make retirement so enjoyable. Thus, mobility is the key to unlocking the most rewarding aspects of your retirement.

Moreover, mobility gives access to involvement and contribution to local communities. It can come in the form of volunteering, participating in nearby organizations or clubs, or even engaging in recreational and cultural events. Being mobile ensures one continues to stay active, have a sense of belonging, and find a purpose in life.

Your physical well-being has close ties with mobility. Navigating freely enables participation in routine physical exercise, which maintains a healthy cardiovascular system, robust bones and muscles, and better control of persistent ailments. Mobility is your gateway to general health.

Let's discuss the complexity of your thought process. Implementing movement in your life has an abundance of advantages for your cognitive abilities. Staying active increases, the supply of oxygen to your brain, decreases the possibility of mental regression, and typically increases your ability to remember details and remain perceptive. Therefore, staying mobile means you're able to keep your mind in excellent working order.

It isn't solely about physical and mental health; it's also concerning the heart. Loss of mobility can induce feelings of loneliness, despondency, and impotence. Conversely, staying dynamic can lead to an elevation of one's temper and better psychological health.

In addition, mobility signifies independence and respectability. It demonstrates one's pride and capacity to make choices about their own life. You have control. You dictate your direction and when to move.

Then there are the personal relationships. With mobility, staying in touch is easier. You can be part of family gatherings, see those special to you, and participate in social activities with ease. It's all about cherishing those deep ties and enhancing your life's overall quality.

Finally, let us not overlook economic independence. Many retirees still desire to function or participate in part-time labor or voluntary jobs during their retirement. Movement is your entry to gaining access to such prospects, benefiting not merely your financial well-being but also your feeling of contentment.

In brief, gaining mobility isn't only about physical movements; it's about incrementing your living standards, cultivating autonomy, and allowing you to maximize your elderly years.

Addressing common challenges in achieving better flexibility and mobility

Let us consider the obstacles some elderly individuals face when augmenting their flexibility and mobility. It is often a difficult mission, and a few common difficulties may be confronted.

As one age, it is common for their muscles and joints to become more rigid. In the morning, you may discover that even tying your shoelaces is more challenging than usual. Thankfully, there is a simple solution to this: be active! You don't need to perform intense exercises; stretching, yoga, and even a bit of tai chi can significantly improve one's flexibility and combat stiffness.

Despite the fear of potential injury that can be off-putting to many, it is entirely understandable to harbor concerns regarding hurting oneself, especially in the early stages. The key to overcoming these anxieties is to move forward at your pace while continuing to take it one step at a time. Chatting with either a medic or a physiotherapist might be beneficial to draw up a specific and secure fitness routine that caters to your individual needs and constraints. With this strategy in place, you will be able to build up your confidence without having to imagine the possibility of suffering an injury.

It is also important to note that persistent health conditions can also be challenging. Ailments such as arthritis can create difficulties. The vital element here is proficiently managing these disorders. Medicines, physiotherapy, and adapting certain lifestyle decisions can help you grapple with the effects of these conditions and encourage better mobility. It may not be simple, but it is definitely beneficial.

Finally, we must discuss motivation. Adhering to your exercise program can be trying, especially when the progress isn't immediate. It's a necessary commitment over the long term. There may be moments when you wish to abandon your efforts. However, uniting with an exercise colleague or taking a group lesson could be an effective way to serve as support. In addition, it's always nice to have someone else to keep you company on your journey. So, while obtaining the desired versatility and agility presents hindrances, with an appropriate plan and some willpower, it's certainly within the realm of possibility.

Chapter 2

Safety Considerations and Precautions

In our quest for improved flexibility and mobility, guaranteeing safety is essential. In this respect, we will explore three essential facets: consulting a medical practitioner, establishing a secure workout location at home, and recognizing accurate warm-up and cool-down techniques.

Consulting a Healthcare Professional Before Starting an Exercise Program

Considering a visit to a medical expert before beginning a fitness program might appear to be an unimportant additional step, but it is, in fact, a crucial action, and let us explore why this is so indispensable.

The Importance of Medical Clearance

Securing medical clearance, akin to receiving a green light from your healthcare provider, is essential to embarking on a sound and successful exercise regimen. Doing so doesn't represent a burdensome necessity but rather the safeguarding of your well-being. Exercise poses different challenges for everyone due to health conditions and circumstances, such as present medical conditions, injuries, and medications, which must be considered before engaging in physical activity.

Imagine you have high blood pressure but are unaware. You plunge into an intensive exercise schedule without contacting a medical expert. The intensive physical strain from the exercise could cause alarming accelerations in your blood pressure, potentially creating grievous health concerns. Furthermore, if you have a joint ailment similar to arthritis, particular exercises may exacerbate the state, leading to pain and discomfort.

By securing medical authorization, you ensure your workout regimen fits your health requirements, realizing the potential threats and doing your best to reduce them. It's about realizing your vulnerabilities and taking the requisite measures to guarantee a harmless and advantageous exercise experience.

Types of Healthcare Professionals to Consult

When deciding who to approach for this important step, your primary care physician is an excellent first point of contact. They exhaustively comprehend your medical background and can evaluate your overall wellness. Speaking with a specialist might be beneficial if you have particular health issues like cardiologic points or musculoskeletal problems. For instance, a cardiac expert can give authoritative counsel if you have heart-related matters, whereas a sports medicine professional can be especially useful when planning a physical exercise-centered schedule.

These experts are outfitted to assess your well-being, grasp your fitness objectives, and recognize potential risks considering your medical history. Consequently, they can recommend workouts that are compatible with your health details.

Your primary care physician particularly functions as the foundation of your healthcare. They can conduct a thorough physical test, analyze your medical record, and factor in attributes such as your age, your existing health condition, and any drugs you may be taking. This exhaustive inspection assists in establishing your base health level and any substantial considerations to be addressed in your exercise plan.

Specialists offer specialized knowledge in particular fields. For example, a cardiologist can be very beneficial if cardiovascular troubles hinder one. This cardiologist might suggest certain drills and their intensity, considering the state of one's heart. In addition, an exercise expert specializing in musculoskeletal health will be pivotal in forming a secure workout routine that meets one's fitness aspirations and cares for their joints and muscles.

Approaching the Conversation

Let us discuss how we can best take on this important conversation with your healthcare provider. This is a partnership; your healthcare provider is your ally in this journey.

Open and honest dialogue is of the utmost importance. Demonstrate your pursuits, whether enhancing flexibility, improving mobility, or all-round welfare. Express your intention to begin an exercise program and talk honestly about any existing health difficulties or past injuries. This openness is essential since your healthcare provider requires this information to form sound judgments.

You'll examine the exercise alternatives that fit your health circumstances during this communication. Your healthcare provider will perform a risk assessment that involves surveying your cardiovascular health, joint health, and any underlying medical concerns. They'll create a customized exercise plan that doesn't only make sure of your safety but also backs your progress toward improved flexibility and mobility.

It's a joint effort, and we encourage your active engagement. Don't hesitate to ask questions or voice any worries you may have. This is your exercise journey, and your healthcare provider is available to ensure it's safe and successful.

Remember, this is not a one-off event. Regular check-ins with your healthcare provider are imperative. These follow-up sessions allow you to monitor your progress and modify your exercise plan as required. Flexibility isn't just about your body but also about your well-being and safety.

Creating a Safe Workout Environment at Home

Having obtained your healthcare provider's approval, you must focus on the location and approach to exercising. The setting of your workout greatly impacts your safety and the efficacy of your routine. Let us take a closer look into creating a safe workout space from the comfort of your own home.

The Importance of a Clutter-Free, Well-Lit Space

Let's say you are locked in your practice session, refining your flexibility and mobility, when you abruptly trip over a dropped object or find it hard to observe your route thanks to lack of lighting. An orderly and well-lit space is both cozy and a safety need.

Clutter can be the main cause of stumbling, and while doing activities that necessitate balance and movement, the last thing you require is an obstacle in your path. Set some time aside to free your exercise space of every likely risk. Ensure the floor is free of items you might step on or slip on.

Suitable lighting is just as important. Clear visibility permits you to keep the right pose during exercises and lessens the probability of any accidents. If your exercise area does not have decent natural light, add extra lighting, such as lamps, to ensure you can watch your actions.

Besides avoiding accidents, illumination also augments your exercise experience. It produces a delightful and motivating atmosphere, which can be useful when finding inspiration to work out is difficult.

Selecting Appropriate Exercise Equipment

Whether relying only on your body weight for your physical activities or using specialized equipment, selecting the proper instruments is fundamental. You must pick what is appropriate for your fitness level and what will enable you to achieve your objectives efficiently and ensure that it remains in great condition.

Utilizing gear like elastic bands, yoga mats, and foam rollers can be incredibly helpful for workouts that mainly strengthen your body's flexibility and mobility. Elastic bands make it easier to adjust the intensity required for stretching exercises, yoga mats give you a comfortable environment for floor exercises, and foam rollers make it simpler to perform self-myofascial release.

If you desire to undertake well-organized and structured strength training, opting for dumbbells or kettlebells is the best option. However, be sure to select weights that match up with your capability level. If you have any doubts, start with the lighter ones, and incrementally increase the resistance as your potential develops.

It is crucial to take care of your exercise equipment. Double-check that your gym gear is in excellent condition, without any loose parts or damage that may cause harm. Regularly assess elastic bands for any hint of harm and make sure that your dumbbells or kettlebells are safe and sturdy.

Properly maintaining your equipment minimizes the risk of incidents while increasing the life expectancy of your exercise devices. This guarantees that your assets in the exercise apparatus will continue to benefit you longer.

Fall Prevention Measures

Falls can be a serious problem, particularly when you're engaged in physical activity. Age makes people more susceptible to incidents of this kind, meaning prevention is paramount. Here are a few steps you can take to reduce the risk of falling:

Secure Rugs: Ensure rugs in the area you're exercising in are firmly in place to reduce the chance of stumbling. Rug grippers or double-sided tape are perfect materials for the job.

Uncluttered Path: Clear any wires, mess, or obstacles from the immediate vicinity to minimize your risk when moving around.

Non-Slip Mats: Under your yoga mat and any exercise equipment, put down non-slip mats that will stay firm even if you sweat heavily during your session.

Supportive Objects: If you're undertaking an activity that requires balance, have something you can hold onto nearby to increase stability and decrease the likelihood of an accident.

Appropriate Footwear: Selecting the correct type of footwear with a good grip is critical. Avoid socks or shoes that may increase the risk of falling.

By adhering to these measures, your chance of an accident during activity should be markedly reduced. Ensure your location is suitably illuminated, debris-free, and outfitted for a safe workout.

Creating and maintaining a safe workout environment is an investment in your physical and mental health. It's important to periodically review your space, ensuring that it is uncluttered and brightly lit, as well as tending to the condition of exercise gear to ensure it is in optimal condition. By prioritizing safety, you can concentrate on developing your agility and mobility in a tranquil and safe atmosphere.

You must strive to improve your mobility and flexibility while continuously prioritizing your safety during exercise. A safe training space is beneficial in safeguarding against potential hazards and helps motivate you and assuage the progress of your fitness mission.

Proper warm-up and cool-down techniques to prevent injury.

Alright! We are about to explore the significance of warming up and cooling down. It isn't merely a fancy ritual; it's a signal from your body that expresses, "Gidday, I'm set to rock and roll!" and "Phew, that was quite strenuous-it's time to rest." Here's why these habits are integral and how you can do them perfectly for enhanced flexibility and movement.

The Warm-Up Dance

Warming up is like the opening scene of an epic show. It establishes the stage, stirs the viewers (your muscles), and ensures a smooth performance. Consider your muscles like rubber bands. When they're cold, they are rigid, and if you try to extend them abruptly, they may break.

This is where warming up comes in. It gradually raises your pulse rate and sends blood to your muscles. This informs your body, "We are about to get going." Nevertheless, that isn't all it does. Here is the scoop on why warming up is a must:

Improved Muscular Function: Before exercising, your muscles loosen gradually. It's as if they are slowly coming out of a long slumber. This is essential to avert any strain on the muscles and guarantee that your movements are buttery-smooth and considered.

Improved Blood Flow: The increased blood flow to the muscles and joints delivers them with oxygen and valuable nutrients. This renders them more power-efficient, primed for action, and less prone to strain.

Mental Preparation: Warming up isn't just a physical event; it's also a mental game. It's your way of transitioning from sleep to intense action. It's your cue to immerse yourself in the activity at hand.

Lessened Risk of Injury: When your muscles are rigid and icy, rushed motions can provoke injury. A warm-up reduces this hazard by gently inflating your body's temperature and flexibility.

Better Range of Motion: Slowly warming up boosts your joint malleability and range of motion. For exercises that target to enhance your flexibility and mobility, this is pure gold.

What should a good warm-up include? It is not simply performing a few jumping jacks. A well-rounded warm-up should entail some aerobic exercises and dynamic stretching. Consider it a mini sequence that adequately gears your body and mentality to tackle the true challenge.

Here's a simple warm-up routine to consider:

Aerobic Exercise: Start with 5-10 minutes of light aerobic exercise. Take a brisk walk, perform stationary cycling, or attempt low-impact aerobics. It's like knocking on the door and announcing, "Let's get active!"

Joint Mobilization: Follow this up with joint mobilization exercises. These are smooth, regulated motions that let your joints move through their total range of motion. You could do shoulder circles, ankle circles, or hip rotations. It's analogous to ringing the bell and signaling, "Time to get to work!"

Dynamic Stretching: Dynamic stretching includes active movements that stretch your muscles and upgrade joint mobility. This might encompass leg swings, arm circles, or trunk rotations. These workouts ready your muscles for the maneuvers you'll do during your workout. It's like a warm-up preceding the actual show.

Right, so that's your pre-workout warm-up. It is akin to preparing your body for the stimulating experience ahead. The issue, though, is that this is not always a matter of universal applicability. It depends on your age, fitness level, and the exercise you will be doing, so your warm-up needs to be tailored. It is all about Customization.

Now you have worked out, and it is time to discuss the cool-down – your grand finale.

The Cool-Down Symphony

The cool-down phase is akin to the curtain call after a tremendous show. It's a chance to transition your body from an energetic state to repose. A properly conducted cool-down brings numerous advantages, some of which are transformative:

Heart Rate Restoration: Your cool-down serves as an occasion for your heart rate to recede to its resting state slowly. This avoids a sudden blood pressure slumping that might otherwise lead to disorientation or fainting. It's like a subtle reminder to your heart that it can unwind now.

Minimized Muscle Soreness: After an exercise session, your muscles may be filled with waste materials such as lactic acid. A cool-down helps wash out these byproducts, thereby cardinally reducing the possibility of muscular soreness. It's similar to tidying up the area after a bash.

Improved Flexibility: As a warm-up enhances flexibility, a cool-down maintains it. Mild, static stretching during the cool-down can help decrease muscle tension and develop your breadth of movement. It's a kind of appreciation for your muscles' hard work.

Mental Relaxation: A cooldown serves as a brief moment of relaxation. It's a period to reflect on your workout, bask in the feelings of accomplishment, and slowly rev up for the normal duties of the day. It's akin to the tranquility that succeeds a storm.

So, what should you encompass in your cool-down routine? It's not merely about slumping on the couch; it's about winding down gracefully.

Stretching: Devote 5-10 minutes to static stretching drills. Focus on the major muscle groups you exerted during your training. Keep each stretch for 15-30 seconds without bouncing. It's like expressing to your muscles, "Good job, now let's unwind."

Deep Breathing: Take a few minutes for deep breathing exercises. Draw in deeply through your nose, permitting your abdomen to rise as you load your lungs with air. Exhale slowly via your mouth. Deep breathing aids soothe your body and mind. It's like the tranquilizing breeze following a storm.

Hydration: Replenish yourself by drinking water. After exertion, you may have lost fluids through sweat, and it's essential to refill them. Appropriate hydration benefits muscle performance and recuperation. It's like giving your body the invigorating drink it deserves.

Recall that your cooldown routine is like the conclusion of a worthy novel. It finals the narration and allows you to feel gratified. Equally to your warm-up, your cooldown should be tailored to what your age, physiques, and capabilities necessitate. It is not something that fits all. It is about ensuring your body acquires the care and consideration it merits.

To briefly summarize the importance of a warm-up and cool-down, these exercises are akin to the backstage and encore for your workout. Much like the bread of a sandwich, they ensure your workout is as optimal as possible. An effective warm-up prepares your body to optimize its physical functioning, reducing the chance of injury and increasing your mobility. Conversely, on completion of your workout regime, a successful cool-down sequence brings your body back to a rested state, allowing your heart rate to recover, decreasing post-workout soreness, and guaranteeing continued flexibility.

It is necessary to remember that this is not just an obligatory step in your workout. Rather, this is an opportunity to perfect your warm-up and cool-down steps to match your needs and desires. It is vital to recognize how your body is responding, and do not hesitate to adjust and trial different techniques until you are content.

Therefore, show your body some love and go out there, do your warm-up, have a fantastic workout, and end it with a meaningful cool-down. You are sure to witness a profound increase in your flexibility and mobility.

Chapter 3

Basic Stretching Exercises for Seniors

Alright, folks, it's time to dive into the world of stretching exercises. Stretching is like giving your body a satisfying yawn – it feels great and keeps your muscles and joints happy. In this chapter, we'll explore some fundamental stretches designed especially for seniors. These exercises are like your daily dose of rejuvenation, helping you maintain and improve your flexibility and mobility.

Neck and Shoulder Stretches

Let's open with one of the most common sources of stress and discomfort for many seniors – the neck and shoulders. The modern lifestyle often encompasses lengthy sitting episodes, whether at a desk, in front of a computer, or while reading a book. This can bring about hunching forward unconsciously, leading to increased tension in the muscles of one's neck and shoulders. This can provoke tightness, uneasiness, and a decrease in flexibility in those regions. But fear not, because the appropriate stretching exercises are helpful in lightening these issues.

Let's commence with a stretch that zeroes in on the sides of your neck, which often becomes particularly tense due to many hours of sitting or any task that necessitates your head to stay stationary. It is known as the "Neck Tilt Stretch." This can be done by sitting in a chair or standing. First, ensure your spine is straight and your feet flat on the ground. To carry out the stretch, easefully tilt your head to one side, taking your ear towards your shoulder. You should sense a gentle stretch along the side of your neck.

As you get accustomed to this pose, keep it for around 15-30 seconds while deeply inhaling and exhaling. When you're done, go back to the original posture and redo the stretch on the opposite side. This effortless exercise can be incredibly beneficial in releasing tension in the sides of your neck and improving your neck's range of motion.

Next, we have the "Neck Rotation Stretch". Much like the preceding exercise, this can be done seated or standing. Start with a straight posture, then turn your neck to the right as far as is comfortable, like you are trying to glance over your shoulder. This movement will give a stretch to the muscles in your neck. Maintain this position for 15 to 30 seconds, taking deep inhalations. Afterward, gradually turn your head to the left side and remain in this stance for the same duration. Doing the Neck Rotation Stretch is great for relieving tension and enhancing the range of motion of your neck.

Our next exercise is the "Shoulder Stretch." This stretch can be a comforting hug to your shoulders and incredibly beneficial if you often have stress or rigidity in this region. To begin, stay upright whether you are seated or standing. Take your right arm across your chest, then use your left hand to attract your right arm nearer to your chest softly. As you do this, you should sense a comfortable stretch in the shoulder area.

Keep in this position for roughly 15 to 30 seconds, and then switch to the left side. It is important to breathe deeply and sink into the stretch. This drill can be especially effective for releasing tightness in the shoulder and enhancing suppleness.

You may wonder how neck and shoulder stretches can increase flexibility and mobility. The answer lies in muscle and joint wellness. When carrying out stretching exercises, we motivate our muscles and joints to work through a broader scope of motion. This helps preserve flexibility and ensures our muscles stay limber. In the case of neck and shoulder stretches, they precisely target spots where we often experience strain due to the necessities of modern life.

The benefits of these stretches extend beyond the physical aspect. Regularly practicing these exercises can bring about your overall well-being by reducing aches, enhancing posture, and lowering the risk of muscle-related injuries. Tension and discomfort in the neck and shoulder area are often caused by prolonged sitting or repetitive movements. Stretching is an effective way to deal with these issues and maintain or improve your range of motion, propagating better flexibility and mobility.

When it comes to making these stretches a regular part of your daily habits, perseverance is essential. All you require is a few minutes every day. These exercises are designed to be straightforward and gentle, so there is no need to take it past your own comfort level. Pay attention to your body and work to raise your flexibility with time incrementally. It's not about attaining a particular degree of flexibility; it's about recognizing the advantages of reduced stress, extended range of motion, and simpler comfort in your neck and shoulders.

In addition, combining these stretches with relaxation methods, for example, deep breathing, can heighten their effectiveness. During these activities, take a few seconds to breathe in and out deeply and relax into the stretches. This mindfulness can alleviate stress and promote a sense of well-being. Therefore, with consistent practice, you should be able to observe these neck and shoulder stretches as reliable allies on your trip toward enhanced flexibility and mobility, eventually leading to a more comfortable and active lifestyle.

Arm and Wrist Stretches

Let's direct our attention away from the upper body and toward another area that frequently experiences pain and strain, especially in age – the arms and wrists. These body parts are true workhorses in our daily activities, from twisting lids off jars to typing out emails or even practicing hobbies like knitting. It's just fair to give them the care and attention they merit.

The arm and wrist extending exercises we'll investigate can aid in preserving flexibility, reducing discomfort, and keeping these areas performing at their best.

Arm Raise Stretch:

Our first stretch is a simple yet powerful exercise for your arms. Get positioned either sitting or standing with your spine upright and your feet firmly placed on the ground. Start by extending your arms in front of yourself at shoulder height. You can have your palms facing down. Now, gradually raise your arms above your head as though trying to reach the ceiling. You might observe a gentle stretch through your arms and shoulders as you do so.

Maintain this extended posture for about 15-30 seconds while you take some deep breaths. Then, slowly lower your arms back down and repeat the exercise as many times as you feel comfortable. You may come to realize that as you increase the repetitions, your arms feel more supple and serene.

The Arm Raise Stretch performs a double purpose. Not only does it elongate your arm muscles, but it additionally assists in bettering your shoulder mobility. This can be especially helpful if you have been noting any stiffness or unease in your shoulders. Additionally, it inspires correct posture, as it opens your chest and shoulders. This can help attain better upper body flexibility and mobility in the long term.

Wrist Flexor Stretch:

The wrists are frequently overlooked when it comes to stretching, yet they play a critical role in our daily activities. The Wrist Flexor Stretch focuses on the muscles on the underside of your lower arm, which control wrist flexion.

To play out this stretch, stretch out your correct arm before you, palm looking down. Utilize your left hand to delicately twist your right wrist so your fingers point towards the floor. As you do this, you will likely encounter a stretch in the underside of your correct lower arm.

Hold this position for around 15-30 seconds, breathing profoundly all through. Repeat this stretch with the left wrist by extending your left arm before you, palm looking down, and using your right hand to twist your left wrist gently.

The Wrist Flexor Stretch has a few advantages that are worth noting. It can help reduce pain or stiffness in the wrists, which is common in older adults. If you have ever encountered wrist pain or discomfort when performing tasks that include gripping, this stretch can be a valuable addition to your day-by-day schedule. Additionally, it bolsters wrist flexibility, making everyday assignments simpler.

Wrist Extensor Stretch:

Let's now turn our attention to the muscles in the upper part of your forearm - your wrist extensors. To perform this stretch, extend your right arm in front of you with your palm upward. Gently use your left hand to bend your right wrist towards the ceiling.

When you do this, you should feel a stretching sensation in the top of your right forearm. Maintain this pose for 15-30 seconds, steadily taking deep breaths the whole time. If you want to focus on your left wrist instead, extend your left arm in such a way with your palm facing up. You should then use your right hand to bend your left wrist.

Similar to the Wrist Flexor Stretch, the Wrist Extensor Stretch supplies you with a range of beneficial outcomes, such as easing any discomfort in your wrists and agreeing your range of movement. This improvement can be priceless if you partake in any tasks that require precise hand and wrist mobility, ranging from cooking to writing to gardening.

So, how do arm and wrist stretches improve flexibility and mobility for seniors? As you age, the muscles and joints gradually lose some of their flexibility, creating stiffness and aches in areas that get lots of use, like the arms and wrists. Engaging in stretching puts those body parts through a more prolonged range of motion. This preserves and boosts their mobility while simultaneously ensuring that the muscles remain pliable, not tightening and restricting.

The advantages of these stretches exceed just physical benefits. They aren't just about flexibility; they also affect overall well-being. Arm and wrist pain caused by regular activities can be reduced by stretching, decreasing any pain, broadening the range of motion, and lessening the risk of muscle-related harm.

Including these stretches in your daily practice is a great way to hold or increase flexibility in your arms and wrists. Just a few minutes each day can make a huge difference. Remember, this isn't about reaching a specified ability of flexibility; it's about benefiting from ease, better range of motion, and higher contentment in your arms and wrists.

Like any different stretching, respect your body and build up your flexibility over time. It's not a competition; it's about caring for yourself. Along with the physical benefits, these stretches can also provide a moment of mindfulness and relaxation, assisting to soothe stress and cultivate a sense of well-being. So, these arm and wrist stretches will grant you relief, suppleness, and general well-being in your day-to-day life.

Lower Back and Spine Stretches

We continue our journey through stretching exercises with a focus on one of the most cardinal sections of our body – the lumbar region, otherwise known as the lower back and spine. These exercise sessions aim to bolster posture, allay unease, and preserve the flexibility of your spine.

The lumbar region is a pivotal part of the body. It holds up the upper body's weight, and it plays an important role in your ability to stand, walk, and maintain good posture. As we age, the muscles and joints in this area can become less flexible and more vulnerable to discomfort. Normal stretching can confront these natural changes and help keep your lower back and spine in a state of maximum performance.

Let us begin with a stretch that peacefully massages your entire spine, the "Cat-Cow Stretch." This sketch is a two-part activity that's habitually employed in yoga and is recognized for its spine-strengthening and suppleness-augmenting advantages.

To begin, position yourself on all fours with your wrists, under your shoulders, and your knees beneath your hips. Keep your back straight and neutral. Take a breath as you arch your back, allowing your stomach to move towards the floor and lifting your head, creating a curve in the lower back. This position is known as the "Cow" pose.

Now exhale as you round your back, tucking your chin towards your chest while engaging your muscles. This is called the "Cat" pose. Flow smoothly between these two positions for around 30 seconds while maintaining steady breaths.

The Cat-Cow Stretch can be compared to giving a soothing massage to your spine. It helps relieve back discomfort and enhances flexibility. This exercise is particularly beneficial for individuals who spend periods sitting or in positions because it promotes fluid movement throughout the spine.

The next exercise is known as the Lower Back Stretch. The Lower Back Stretch can be done while seated on a chair with your feet resting firmly on the ground. This move is particularly beneficial for people who struggle with stiffness or pain in the lower back and hip area. To do this, position your right ankle on top of your left knee, using a gentle press to bring the right knee closer to the floor. Remain in this stance for 15-30 seconds, breathing deeply as you relax in order to gain the full benefits of the stretch. Once you're done, switch to the other side by placing your left ankle atop your right knee and pushing the left knee in the same manner.

The Spinal Twist is another stretching exercise that can be done while seated in a chair with your feet flatly planted on the floor. It is designed to enhance your spine's range of motion. To do so, sit straight and keep your knees pointing forward. Slowly twist your upper body to the right, using your left arm to anchor yourself to the back of the chair and using your right hand to apply pressure to your right thigh, deepening the twist. Maintain this placement for 15-30 seconds, focusing on your breaths. Then, switch to the left side.

These lower back and spine stretches are highly beneficial for seniors, strengthening their flexibility, range of motion, and overall energy. This is especially helpful for those who often feel discomfort when sitting for extended periods. Plus, these exercises not only improve physical comfort but also mental well-being, promoting relaxation and easing stress.

A few minutes of stretches each day can give seniors an abundance of advantages. Patience is important; we should never push our body beyond its limits. It's a journey of taking care of oneself, not a race. With regular practice, these stomach and back stretches can provide comfort, agility, and a sense of calm within the everyday.

Chapter 4

Gentle Full-Body Stretching

Routine

In the pursuit of maintaining a healthy, lively lifestyle as a senior, the significance of a balanced, overall full-body stretching regimen simply cannot be diminutive. This section will guide you through a far-reaching stretching practice that considers every major muscle group from the skull to the feet. By engaging in this routine, you will be augmenting flexibility, boosting mobility, and nurturing your all-round state of well-being.

Head-to-Toe Stretching

Let's delve into the heart of our full-body stretching routine, starting with the invigorating head-to-toe stretches. Picture this: you've just woken up, or maybe you're taking a break from your day's activities. It's the perfect moment to give your body the gift of stretching.

Neck Stretch:

Our journey begins with a gentle, nurturing neck stretch. Consider your neck to be a link between your head and the rest of your body. It serves as an essential link between your brain and the outside environment. This bridge may begin to feel a little rickety and rusted over time. This is where this stretch comes into play.

Make sure you're in a comfortable sitting or standing position before you begin. Take a long breath in and slowly tilt your head to the right as you exhale, bringing your ear closer to your shoulder. A mild stretch should be felt on the left side of your neck.

The important thing to remember here is to walk gently and deliberately. There's no need to rush. Your body appreciates the time you put into taking care of it. Continue to take slow, deep breaths while holding this posture for around 15-30 seconds. It's as if you're telling your neck, "I'm here, and I'm taking care of you."

Return your attention to the center and notice the subtle release of tension on the left side of your neck. And now for the magic: repeat on the opposite side. Tilt your head to the left and bring your ear close to your shoulder. Hold for another 15-30 seconds, being sure you breathe deeply and evenly.

The neck stretch serves as a soothing balm for the tensions of everyday life. If you spend long hours sitting, working on a computer, or reading, this stretch is your way of telling your neck, "I understand your struggles, and I'm here to make you feel better."

Arm Stretch:

Arm stretches are the next step in our journey. Consider your arms to be your everyday assistants. They reach for items on high shelves, carry grocery bags, and offer consoling embraces. They are there for you every day, therefore it's only reasonable that you take care of them.

You can sit or stand for this stretch, whatever is more comfortable for you. To begin, ensure that your spine is straight and that your feet are flat on the ground. Take a deep breath and appreciate the life in your arms. Extend your arms straight out in front of you at shoulder height, palms facing down. It's as if you're greeting your arms and recognizing their significance.

Then, gradually lift your arms upwards, reaching towards the ceiling. Feel the slight stretch in your arms and shoulders as you perform this. This stretch is like a warm embrace for your arms, thanking them for everything they do every day.

Hold this position for 15-30 seconds while breathing deeply. You may then drop your arms and enjoy the feeling of freedom. This practice can be repeated as many times as you desire. It's your way of saying, "Arms, I appreciate everything you do for me."

The arm stretch is particularly beneficial for maintaining flexibility and comfort in your upper body. It's like a sigh of relief for your shoulders, which often bear the weight of the day's activities. With each repetition of this stretch, you're helping your arms maintain their range of motion, promoting better posture, and reducing discomfort.

Back Stretch:

Let's get to the back stretch now. Your back serves as the core pillar that keeps you upright. It is essential to your posture, balance, and general health. Unfortunately, it can also cause discomfort, especially as we become older. This is when the back stretch comes in handy.

You may perform this one standing or sitting, whichever seems more comfortable for you. First, make sure your spine is straight and your feet are solidly grounded. Allow your breath to flow freely, like a calm stream.

Reach your right arm across your chest to the left side, as if you were hugging yourself. Feel the back extend and the gentle opening of your chest. Continue to take deep breaths while holding this posture for around 15-30 seconds.

Now, relax your right arm and feel the comfort in your back and chest. And, of course, it's time for the other side. Extend your left arm across your chest to the right side, as if hugging yourself again. Feel the stretch and allow your breath to flow freely as you hold this position for around 15-30 seconds.

The back stretch feels like a warm hug for your spine and chest. It's an expression of gratitude for all they do to keep you upright and mobile. This stretch can help you improve your posture, relieve pain, and relax your back and chest muscles.

Hip Stretch:

Let us now shift our attention to your hips. Your hip muscles are essential in all of your daily activities, from walking to sitting. They are the unsung heroes who allow you to stay mobile, and they, like all heroes, require some attention.

You may do this stretch while sitting or standing, depending on what feels best for you. Make sure your spine is straight and your feet are firmly grounded. Take a few deep breaths and concentrate on your hips.

Tilt your right hip to the right and feel the strain on your left side. Hold this position for 15-30 seconds, taking deep breaths throughout.

Feel the gentle relaxation of tension on your left side as you release your right hip. And now it's time for the other side. Feel the stretch on your right side by tilting your left hip to the left. Hold this position for 15-30 seconds while breathing deeply and evenly.

The hip stretch is a gentle way of saying thank you to your hip muscles. It's a method of acknowledging their value in your life and ensuring that they stay flexible and helpful. This stretch can help relieve hip pain, increase flexibility, and improve general mobility.

Leg Stretch:

Our adventure continues with the legs, which serve as the foundation for your mobility. Your legs are your closest companions whether you're strolling around the park, climbing stairs, or even dancing.

This stretch may be done sitting or standing, depending on your preference. Begin by making sure your spine is straight and your feet are solidly grounded. Feel your body's connection to the earth underneath you.

Extend your right leg in front of you, toes pointing upwards. You should feel a slight stretch in your calf and the back of your leg as you execute this. Hold this posture for 15-30 seconds, breathing deeply to accompany the stretch.

Relax your right leg and enjoy the sensation of relaxation. And, you guessed it, it's time for the other side. Extend your left leg in front of you, toes pointing upward. Feel the slight stretch in your left calf and the back of your left leg as you do this. Hold this position for 15-30 seconds while breathing deeply and evenly.

The leg stretch is a way of saying "thank you" to your legs. It's your method of showing your appreciation for their contribution to your everyday activities and ensuring they stay adaptable and supportive. This stretch can help to relieve pain, increase leg flexibility, and encourage pleasant mobility.

Foot Stretch:

Lastly, we arrive at your feet. Your feet are the unsung heroes of your mobility. They carry you through life, one step at a time. Let us shower them with affection.

This stretch may be done while sitting. Begin by keeping your spine straight and your feet firmly planted. Take a few deep breaths and concentrate on your feet.

Extend your right leg in front of you softly, keeping your heel on the ground. Extend your toes toward your shin. You should feel a stretch on the underneath of your foot when you do this. Hold this posture for about 15-30 seconds, breathing deeply and evenly.

Feel the gentle relaxation as you release your right foot. It's time to put the other foot forward. Extend your left leg out in front of you, heel on the ground. Stretch the underside of your left foot by flexing your toes upward toward your shin. Hold this position for 15-30 seconds while breathing deeply and evenly.

The foot stretch is a way of saying "thank you" to your feet for their unending support. Stretching your feet relieves discomfort, promotes flexibility, and improves general stability and support.

This stretching routine from head to toe is a healing gift to your body. It's about pausing to recognize and care for every part of yourself, from your neck to your toes. By following this complete practice daily, you will invest in improved flexibility, mobility, and a greater sense of well-being. So, remember this practice the next time you start your day or take a break from your everyday duties. It's your chance to nourish your body and improve the quality of your life, one stretch at a time.

Emphasizing Slow and Controlled Movements

As we journey through our full-body stretching routine, there's an essential aspect we'd like to highlight - the emphasis on slow and controlled movements. This component is about mindfulness, understanding your body, and savoring the stretching experience.

Consider yourself on a leisurely stroll around a peaceful park. The sun is warm on your skin, while a light wind rustles the tree leaves. You walk slowly, taking in the beauty of your surroundings and allowing the moment's pleasures to wash over you. This is similar to the aim of slow and controlled movements in stretching.

We routinely hurry through things, including exercise, in today's fast-paced society. Stretching, on the other hand, provides a unique chance to slow down, pay attention to your body, and connect with it on a deeper level. It's time to take care of your physical and emotional health.

Why Slow and Controlled Movements Matter:

- Safety: First and foremost, slow, and controlled movements are safe. When you rush through stretches with sudden, jerky motions, you risk overstretching, straining your muscles, or even injuring yourself. By taking your time, you're being kind to your body and ensuring it's safe from harm.

- Mind-Body Connection: Slow and controlled movements allow you to build a strong mind-body connection. This means that you're not just going through the motions; you're actively engaging with your body, feeling each stretch, and understanding your body's unique needs. This connection can be incredibly empowering and can extend beyond your stretching routine into other areas of your life.

- Tension Release: Rushing through stretches can actually increase tension in your muscles. On the other hand, slow and controlled movements promote the release of tension. Think of it as coaxing your muscles into relaxation. This not only feels fantastic but also contributes to improved flexibility.

- Stress Reduction: Fast, hurried movements can be stressful for both your body and your mind. In contrast, slow and controlled movements have a calming effect. They can serve as a meditative practice, reducing stress and promoting a sense of peace and mindfulness.

- Better Results: When you stretch slowly and deliberately, you'll find that you achieve better results. Your muscles and connective tissues respond more effectively to the stretch, elongating and releasing tension. This ultimately leads to improved flexibility and reduced muscle tightness.

The Power of Your Breath:

Let's speak about the power of your breath to truly embrace slow and controlled movements. Your breath is a tool that may help you connect with your body and make your stretches more effective.

Imagine you are in the middle of a stretch. Take a deep breath, filling your lungs completely, as you go into the stretch. Feel your body lengthen as it stretches. Imagine releasing tension and letting your body to settle into the stretch as you exhale.

For instance, during the arm stretch, take a deep breath in as you raise your arms overhead, feeling the stretch in your arms and shoulders. Allow your body to relax into the stretch as you exhale, reaching a bit further. This coordinated breathing and stretching is reminiscent of a dance between your body and your breath.

Let's Put It Into Practice:

Assume you're performing a back stretch. Inhale deeply as you gently reach your right arm across your chest to the left side. Feel your chest opening and stretching. Allow your body to relax into the stretch a little more as you exhale. This gentle, synchronized movement and breath allow your body to release stress one inch at a time.

It is not a race; rather, it is a journey. A path toward a more relaxed, flexible, and mindful you. Slow and controlled movements require you to take your time, relish each stretch, and understand your body's unique responses.

Incorporating Mindfulness:

Mindfulness is an integral part of slow and controlled movements. It means being fully present in the moment, observing your body's sensations, and letting go of distractions. It's about being kind to yourself, acknowledging your limitations, and appreciating your progress.

Picture this: You're doing the hip stretch. As you tilt your right hip to the right, take a moment to close your eyes if that's comfortable for you. Focus on the sensation in your left hip. What does it feel like? Is there tension? Can you feel it slowly releasing as you hold the stretch? Are you breathing deeply and evenly?

This level of attention and awareness is what mindfulness is all about. It's your chance to nurture your body, clear your mind, and release the tensions of the day.

Enjoying the Journey:

We focus on the journey rather than the destination (the completed stretch) in our full-body stretching practice. Each stretch is a unique experience, and each repetition may bring something fresh to the table. It's not about rushing to the finish line; it's about enjoying the journey.

When you take the time to move slowly and deliberately, you're offering your body the gift of self-care. You are taking care of yourself, both physically and mentally. This can be a priceless gesture of self-love in today's fast-paced world.

So, as you continue your stretching exercise, keep in mind the need of slow, controlled movements. Take in every stretch, every breath, and every moment. It's your chance to strengthen your mind-body connection, release tension, reduce stress, and achieve greater results. Take advantage of this opportunity to become a more calm, flexible, and mindful version of yourself.

Holding Stretches for an Appropriate Duration

We've started our full-body stretching regimen, stressing slow and controlled movements. Now, let's look at the importance of holding stretches for a suitable amount of time. This section is similar to the encore of a beautiful musical performance; it is where the magic happens.

Have you ever raced through a task only to realize you overlooked something crucial? Stretching is similar in that sense. It's not just about the stretch, but also about how long you stay in that stretched position. Let's look at why holding stretches is important and how to get the most out of them.

The Science of Stretching:

Let's start with the why before we get into the how. Stretching your neck, arms, back, hips, legs, or feet essentially stretches your muscles and connective tissues. This lengthening is necessary for maintaining and developing flexibility.

Our muscles and connective tissues function similarly to elastic bands. They can get tighter, shorter, and less flexible over time, especially as we age. Stretching is vital because it helps restore and maintain the natural flexibility of these tissues.

When you stretch a muscle or a set of muscles, your brain sends a signal to them to relax. The longer you hold the stretch, the deeper the relaxation. It's like a muscle sighing with relaxation, gradually releasing its tension.

Consider a rubber band that has been tightly twisted. When you carefully release it, it unwinds gently while retaining its integrity. But if you release off too quickly, it snaps back to its former shape. The same idea applies to your muscles; holding a stretch for a longer period of time allows your muscles to relax more effectively, allowing you to experience a deeper and more lasting stretch.

Holding Stretches for Flexibility:

Holding a stretch for a suitable amount of time essentially trains your muscles to accommodate a broader range of motion. This expanded range of motion leads to increased flexibility, which improves overall mobility.

Flexibility is important for a multitude of reasons, including bending to tie your shoelaces, reaching for objects on high shelves, and simply moving freely and pleasantly. The longer you hold a stretch, the more your muscles and connective tissues are encouraged to stay supple and allow you to move freely.

Relief from Muscle Tension:

Holding a stretch is like to applying a soothing balm to your muscles. Stretching can provide relief from muscle stress or stiffness caused by a long day at work or physical activity.

For example, during the arm stretch, as you raise your arms overhead and hold that position, you're allowing your arm muscles to relax. You may experience a pleasant sense of relaxation as the tightness in your shoulders gradually dissipates.

Similarly, during the leg stretch, as you extend and hold your right leg, you are providing comfort to the muscles in your calf and back of your thigh. You may experience a gradual release of tension in your leg, making it feel more relaxed and comfortable.

Mental Relaxation:

The act of holding a stretch offers both physical and mental advantages. It's a meditative exercise, a focused moment in your day. You can use this time to clear your mind, focus on your breath, and release stress while maintaining a stretch.

Let's go over the back stretch again. You're not simply extending your muscles when you reach your right arm across your chest to the left side and hold that position; you're also having a relaxing sensation. Your body and mind are cooperating to relieve tension, both physically and mentally.

It's during this time that you can take a few deep breaths, close your eyes if you wish, and immerse yourself in the sensation of the stretch. This mental relaxation can be as beneficial as the physical aspect of stretching.

How Long Should You Hold a Stretch?

"How long should I hold a stretch?" the question arises. The answer will differ based on your body and the stretch you're practicing. In general, holding a stretch for 15-30 seconds is a good point to start. However, there are no hard and fast rules, and you should be guided by your comfort and progress.

As a general rule, aim for at least 15 seconds and progressively go to 30 seconds or more if you feel comfortable. If you experience any discomfort or pain, you must quickly release the stretch. The idea is to feel a gentle, tension-releasing stretch rather than to push your body past its limits.

Exploring the Experience:

Each stretch in our full-body practice gives you a unique opportunity to experiment with holding a stretch. Take note of how your body reacts while you hold the stretch. Is there a gradual release of tension? Can you feel your muscles and connective tissues responding to the stretch and allowing you to move a little bit further?

Pay attention to your calf and the back of your thigh as you extend your left leg in front of you and hold it. Take note of how the muscles gradually relax. It's as if your body and the stretch are having a conversation, with both sides listening and responding.

The Importance of Breathing:

In this journey of holding stretches, your breath is an invaluable companion. It's more than just a physiological process; it's a technique that may help you connect with your body and make your stretches more effective.

Take, for example, the backstretch. Inhale deeply as you reach your right arm across your chest to the left side. Feel your chest opening and stretching. Allow your body to relax into the stretch even more as you exhale. Your breath acts as the orchestra's director, guiding the entire experience.

Breathing deeply and evenly during a stretch is a simple yet powerful technique. It reduces discomfort, enhances relaxation, and allows your muscles to respond more effectively to the stretch.

Reflecting on Progress:

It's important to reflect on your success in holding stretches as you continue your stretching routine. You may discover that you can hold stretches for longer periods of time or that the sensation of tension release gets more pronounced over time.

The leg stretch is an excellent example. As you hold the stretch and extend your right leg, you may notice that your calf and back of your thigh get more flexible with practice. You may be able to hold the stretch for a longer period of time, and your sense of relaxation may deepen.

This reflection on progress is a motivating factor in your stretching journey. It's a reminder that by dedicating time to your body, you're not only maintaining your flexibility and mobility but also making gradual improvements.

Enjoy the Journey:

Holding stretches for an appropriate duration is about enjoying the journey. It's your chance to nurture your body, release tension, increase flexibility, and savor the experience of stretching. In a world that often rushes, this practice allows you to slow down, connect with your body, and be present in the moment.

So, as you continue your full-body stretching routine, remember that holding a stretch is like having a conversation with your body. It's about listening, responding, and nurturing your physical and mental well-being. It's not just about the stretch; it's about the time you spend in that stretched position, allowing your body to release tension and experience a sense of freedom and ease. Enjoy this journey toward improved flexibility, reduced muscle tension, and enhanced mindfulness.

Chapter 5

Chair-based Stretching and

Mobility Exercises

In this chapter, we will explore a series of chair-based stretching and mobility exercises designed to enhance flexibility, reduce tension, and improve overall well-being. These exercises are tailored to be accessible for seniors of all mobility levels and can be comfortably performed in the familiar setting of your home.

Seated Neck and Shoulder Rolls: Relieving Tension and Promoting Relaxation

Let us start with a simple but effective exercise: seated neck and shoulder rolls. Imagine a peaceful moment. You're sitting in a strong chair, your feet firmly planted on the ground, and your back is gently supported. Your neck and shoulders, two frequently overlooked body parts, have been tense. It's a common scenario in our modern life, with activities that strain these vital body components. Seated neck and shoulder rolls are the key to gently releasing this tension.

It is impossible to overestimate the importance of neck and shoulder relief. These areas take the brunt of our daily activities, whether they are hours spent typing on a computer or the physical demands of daily living. Unresolved tension can cause pain, reduced mobility, and even migraines. Seated neck and shoulder rolls are an easy yet effective remedy to this condition.

How to Perform Seated Neck and Shoulder Rolls:

1. Begin by sitting comfortably in the chair with your feet flat on the ground.

2. Close your eyes, if you wish, to enhance your focus on the exercise.

3. Inhale deeply, allowing your chest to rise as you fill your lungs with air.

4. As you exhale, gently drop your chin to your chest, feeling a stretch in the back of your neck. Hold this position for a moment.

5. Slowly roll your head to the right, moving your right ear towards your right shoulder. Hold this stretch for a few seconds.

6. Continue the circular motion by rolling your head back and tilting your left ear towards your left shoulder.

7. Complete the circle by rolling your head to the front again, returning your chin to your chest.

8. Repeat this circular motion for about 30 seconds, then reverse the direction, rolling your head to the left.

9. After completing the reverse circle, return your head to the center and take a few deep breaths.

10. Roll your shoulders in a gentle circular motion, bringing them forward, up, back, and down. This helps to release tension in the shoulder area.

11. After about 30 seconds of shoulder rolls, reverse the direction, moving your shoulders in the opposite circle.

12. Finish by bringing your shoulders to a relaxed, neutral position.

The exercise begins with a gentle tension release. It's as if your neck receives a loving cuddle when you bow your chin towards your chest. The stretch around the back of your neck starts to untangle the knots of stress that have built up. When you begin the circular motion by moving your head to the right, it feels like you're getting a relaxing massage for your neck and shoulders. With each circle, your muscles can sigh in relief because of this motion's methodical, slow tempo. Turning your head to the left ensures that both sides of your neck and shoulders receive equal attention and relief.

During this activity, your breath is really important. Deep, deliberate breathing improves the practice's effectiveness. Deep breathing oxygenates your body, supplying nutrition to your muscles and tissues. This allows your muscles to relax more completely throughout the stretch. Exhaling not only releases air but also tension. It's as if you're breathing a sigh of relief, enabling your body to sink deeper into the stretch.

Seated neck and shoulder rolls are more than just a physical exercise; they are also a type of mindfulness. It is recommended that you close your eyes for this exercise if you feel comfortable doing so. This simple act draws your focus inward, allowing you to be acutely aware of your body's sensations. This mindfulness serves as a moment of mental relaxation, providing a little break from the everyday grind.

Stress often has an adverse effect on our bodies, and the neck and shoulders are common areas for stress to appear physically. We stiffen when stressed, which can contribute to chronic tension. Seated neck and shoulder rolls release accumulated stress and the weight it places on your shoulders.

This workout also improves flexibility and mobility. You gradually extend the range of motion in your neck and shoulders with each circular motion. This increased flexibility translates into more comfort and ease in your daily tasks, such as rotating your head more freely, reaching for products on high shelves without strain, and maintaining good posture.

The convenience of seated neck and shoulder rolls is unrivaled. This workout may be done almost anywhere. All you need is a chair whether you're at your workplace, in your living room, or even outside. Consider making this workout a part of your regular regimen. It can be a wonderful break during a long job, a relaxing moment before night, or a small intermission between your everyday tasks. It's crucial to remember that these exercises aren't one-size-fits-all; you can tailor the experience to your specific requirements. If you feel that turning your head in one direction for 30 seconds is too long, start with a lesser duration and progressively increase it.

Ankle and Foot Stretches Using a Chair: Enhancing Mobility from the Ground Up

The foundation of our mobility is our feet. We move more easily and comfortably when our ankles and feet are flexible and strong. Chair exercises for the ankles and feet help to improve flexibility, reduce stiffness, and promote mobility in these important body regions.

Begin by imagining your feet flat on the earth, providing a solid, stable base. Your feet and ankles play an important role in your daily activities. They are constantly at work whether you are walking, standing, or sitting.

Foot and ankle stiffness and soreness can develop over time. Various circumstances, such as aging, inactivity, or specific medical disorders can cause this. The good news is that these stretches can help with pain relief.

How to Perform Ankle and Foot Stretches Using a Chair:

1. Begin by sitting in a sturdy chair with your feet flat on the ground, hip-width apart.

2. Inhale deeply, lengthening your spine.

3. As you exhale, raise your right foot slightly off the ground.

4. With your right foot hovering, flex and point your toes several times. This movement helps to maintain flexibility in your ankle.

5. Rotate your right foot at the ankle, moving it in a circular motion for about 30 seconds in each direction.

6. Lower your right foot to the ground.

7. Repeat the same sequence with your left foot.

8. After completing both feet, you can take a moment to gently roll your ankles by making circular motions with your feet. This further promotes flexibility in the ankle joint.

These ankle and foot stretches can significantly improve your feet and ankles' mobility and flexibility. You can relieve discomfort and prevent the danger of stiffness in certain areas by completing them regularly. Furthermore, keeping your feet and ankles flexible can help you retain your balance and lower your chance of falling, which is especially important for seniors.

As with any activity, listening to your body and avoiding overexertion is critical. Stop and consult a healthcare expert if you encounter pain or discomfort while executing these stretches. Your safety and comfort should always come first.

Seated Spinal Twists and Stretches:

Nurturing Spinal Health

Our spine serves as our primary support system. It is essential for maintaining proper posture, balance, and mobility. However, the spine can stiffen as we age, causing discomfort and a loss of movement. Seated spinal twists and stretches are exercises that promote spinal flexibility and wellness.

These exercises target the lumbar (lower back), thoracic (upper and middle back), and cervical (neck) portions of the spine. They consist of moderate twisting and stretching movements that help relieve stress, promote flexibility, and lower the risk of back pain. Let's look at how to do seated spinal twists and stretches.

How to Perform Seated Spinal Twists and Stretches:

1. Begin by sitting in a sturdy chair with your feet flat on the ground, hip-width apart.

2. Inhale deeply, lengthening your spine and ensuring upright posture.

3. As you exhale, gently twist your upper body to the right. Place your right hand outside your left knee for support, and your left hand can rest on the chair's armrest.

4. Hold the twist for 15-30 seconds while breathing deeply and comfortably.

5. Inhale as you return to the center.

6. Exhale and twist your upper body to the left, following the same steps.

7. Hold the twist for 15-30 seconds while maintaining deep, relaxed breathing.

8. Inhale as you return to the center.

To increase the effectiveness of these seated spinal twists and stretches, repeat them many times on each side. They are a gentle yet effective approach to preserve spine health and enhance back flexibility.

Seated Leg Stretches for Hips and Hamstrings: Supporting Lower Body Flexibility

Our legs, especially our hips and hamstrings, are critical to our mobility and overall physical comfort. These areas, however, are prone to stiffness, which can limit our range of motion and possibly cause discomfort and pain. Seated leg stretches with a chair are intended to target the hips and hamstrings, increasing flexibility and comfort in these important areas.

How to Perform Seated Leg Stretches:

1. Start by sitting in a sturdy chair with your back well-supported and feet flat on the ground.

2. Extend your right leg in front of you, keeping your knee straight but not locked.

3. Inhale deeply, lengthening your spine.

4. As you exhale, gently lean forward from your hips, reaching toward your toes. You can rest your hands on your thigh or shin, or if possible, try to reach your toes. Go only as far as your flexibility allows without causing discomfort.

5. Hold the stretch for 15-30 seconds, continuing to breathe deeply and comfortably.

6. Inhale as you return to an upright position.

7. Repeat the same sequence with your left leg.

Performing these seated leg stretches regularly can enhance the flexibility and comfort of your hips and hamstrings. It's essential to listen to your body and avoid pushing yourself too hard. If you experience pain or discomfort during the stretches, stop and consult with a healthcare professional if necessary.

Maintaining flexibility in your lower body is crucial for activities like getting in and out of chairs, walking, and even bending to pick up items. These stretches can contribute to a more comfortable and mobile lifestyle.

Incorporating these chair-based stretching and mobility exercises into your daily routine can help enhance your overall well-being. Remember to perform these exercises at your own pace and within your comfort level. The goal is not to force your body into challenging positions but to gently promote flexibility, relieve tension, and increase mobility. As with any new exercise routine, if you have existing medical conditions or concerns, it's advisable to consult with a healthcare professional before starting. Your well-being should always be the top priority.

Chapter 6

Floor-based stretching and

Mobility Exercises

In this chapter, we delve into a series of floor-based stretching and mobility exercises that can contribute to your flexibility, alleviate tension, and promote a sense of relaxation. These exercises offer a different dimension to your flexibility routine and can be particularly beneficial if you are comfortable getting down to the floor.

Supine Hamstring Stretches: Unwinding the Back of the Legs

The hamstrings are a collection of three muscles on the back of your thigh, including the biceps femoris, semitendinosus, and semimembranosus. Because these muscles are essential for the movement of your hip and knee joints, they are crucial for numerous daily tasks such as walking, jogging, and bending. However, as we get older, our hamstrings might become tight and less flexible. This tightness can cause pain, a reduced range of motion, and an increased risk of injury. Supine hamstring stretches are a great technique to increase the flexibility of these important muscles, relieve tension, and promote relaxation.

Understanding the Hamstrings:

Before we get into how to do supine hamstring stretches, it's important to understand the role of the hamstrings in your body. The hamstring muscles control the flexion and extension of your knees and hips. These movements are essential in daily tasks such as walking, jogging, and rising from a seated position. These activities are more pleasant and efficient when your hamstrings are flexible and well-maintained.

However, the hamstrings are prone to tightening and shortening with time, which can have several consequences. They can restrict your range of motion when they tighten, making actions like bending over to tie your shoes or reaching for items on high shelves more difficult. Tight hamstrings may increase the risk of strain or injury, especially during activities that demand quick movements or stretching.

How to Perform Supine Hamstring Stretches:

Let's dive into how to perform supine hamstring stretches:

1. **Find a Comfortable Surface**: To begin, locate a comfortable surface to lie on, such as a yoga mat or a carpeted floor. Alternatively, you can perform these stretches on a bed if you find it more comfortable.

2. **Lie on Your Back**: Position yourself on your back with your legs extended fully along the floor. Keep your arms relaxed by your sides.

3. **Focus on Your Breath**: Take a moment to connect with your breath. Inhale deeply, feeling your chest and abdomen rise. As you exhale, release any tension you may be holding in your body. Deep, controlled breathing is essential during these stretches as it aids in relaxation and muscle release.

4. **Bend One Knee**: Bend one of your knees, bringing it toward your chest while extending the other leg fully along the floor. This is the starting position for the stretch.

5. **Clasp Your Hands**: Gently clasp your hands behind your thigh, just below your knee. If you find it challenging to reach your thigh comfortably, you can use a towel or a yoga strap to assist you.

6. **Straighten Your Leg**: With a straight spine and a relaxed neck, gently straighten your bent leg while keeping your hands clasped behind your thigh. As you extend your leg, you'll feel the stretch in the back of your thigh, in the hamstring muscles. Go only as far as your flexibility allows without causing discomfort. It's crucial to note that you may be unable to straighten your leg fully, and that's perfectly fine. The goal is to feel a gentle stretch, not to force your leg straight.

7. **Hold the Stretch**: Once you've reached a comfortable point in the stretch, hold this position for 15-30 seconds. Continue to breathe deeply and comfortably while in the stretched position.

8. **Release Your Leg**: Slowly release your leg and return it to the floor.

9. **Repeat with the Other Leg**: After completing the stretch with one leg, repeat the same sequence with your other leg.

Incorporating these supine hamstring stretches into your everyday routine can dramatically improve your flexibility and overall well-being. By doing them consciously and consistently, you will not only improve your physical comfort but also enjoy a deeper sense of inner calm and relaxation. These stretches may be done at home or nearly anywhere, making them an adaptable addition to your regular routine.

Remember to invest in your physical and mental well-being the next time you do these supine hamstring stretches. Enjoy the sense of relaxation and tranquility that comes with each breath as you stretch your hamstrings and release tension. These stretches will help you on your way to greater flexibility and mobility, supporting your active and joyful lifestyle.

Seated and Supine Hip Flexor Stretches: Improving Hip Mobility

Hip flexors are a set of muscles in the front of your hips and upper thighs. These muscles are required for various activities such as walking, running, climbing stairs, and standing up from a seated position. As we age, our hip flexors tend to tighten, limiting our range of motion, causing discomfort, and affecting our overall mobility. Hip flexor stretches, both seated and supine, are an effective technique to improve the mobility of these important muscles, resulting in increased comfort and ease in daily activities.

Understanding the Hip Flexors:

Before we explore how to do seated and supine hip flexor stretches, it's important to understand the importance of hip flexor muscles in your body. The primary hip flexor muscles are the iliopsoas, rectus femoris, and sartorius. These muscles are essential for hip and thigh mobility, specifically flexion of the hip joint and extension of the knee joint.

The hip flexors are engaged every time you take a step, climb stairs, or elevate your legs. However, with age and prolonged sitting, these muscles can become tight and less flexible, causing discomfort and reduced range of motion, and perhaps affecting your gait.

How to Perform Seated and Supine Hip Flexor Stretches:

Let's explore how to perform seated and supine hip flexor stretches effectively:

Seated Hip Flexor Stretch:

1. Start by sitting on the floor with your legs extended in front of you.

2. Bend one knee and place your foot flat on the floor.

3. Bring your opposite ankle to rest on the thigh of your bent leg, just above your knee.

4. Inhale deeply and lengthen your spine.

5. As you exhale, gently lean forward toward your foot while keeping your back straight. You should feel the stretch in the hip and thigh of your bent leg.

6. Hold this stretch for 15-30 seconds while breathing deeply and relaxing.

7. Inhale as you return to an upright position.

8. Repeat the same sequence with your other leg.

Supine Hip Flexor Stretch:

1. Lie on your back with your legs extended.

2. Bend one knee and bring it toward your chest.

3. Clasp your hands behind your thigh, just below your knee.

4. Gently pull your knee toward your chest to feel the stretch in your hip and thigh.

5. Hold this stretch for 15-30 seconds.

6. Inhale deeply and release your leg.

7. Repeat the same sequence with your other leg.

These seated and supine hip flexor exercises help improve the mobility and comfort of your hip and thigh muscles. You will enjoy enhanced physical well-being and a greater sensation of relaxation if you practice them thoughtfully and consistently. These stretches may be done at home or anywhere, making them a versatile addition to your regular routine.

Enjoy the sense of relaxation and serenity that comes with each breath as you stretch your hip flexors and release tension. These stretches will help you on your journey to greater flexibility and mobility, supporting your active and joyful lifestyle.

Quadratus Lumborum Stretch: Easing Lower Back Discomfort

The quadratus lumborum, commonly called the QL, is a deep muscle in the lower back. It is important in motions involving the lumbar spine, pelvis, and ribs. This muscle helps with various activities, such as bending to the side, standing, walking, and even breathing. However, the QL can become tight and less flexible as we age, resulting in discomfort, restricted range of motion, and probable lower back pain. Stretching the quadratus lumborum is an effective approach to target this muscle, increase its flexibility, and provide lower back pain relief.

Understanding the Quadratus Lumborum:

Before we dive into how to perform QL stretches, it's essential to comprehend the significance of the quadratus lumborum muscle in your body. The QL muscles run on both sides of your spine, connecting your pelvis to your lowest rib and lumbar vertebrae. These muscles enable you to perform various movements, such as bending to the side, twisting your torso, and maintaining an upright posture.

The QL is in charge of stabilizing the lower back, and when it is flexible and well-maintained, it helps you move freely and comfortably. However, due to factors such as prolonged sitting or aging, the QL can become stiff, causing lower back discomfort and limited mobility.

How to Perform Quadratus Lumborum Stretches:

Let's explore how to perform quadratus lumborum stretches effectively:

Seated Quadratus Lumborum Stretch:

1. Begin by sitting on the floor with your legs extended in front of you.

2. Bend your right knee and place your foot on the floor, with your heel positioned close to your right buttock.

3. Cross your left leg over your right, placing your left foot on the floor outside of your right knee. Your left knee should be bent, and your left foot flat on the floor.

4. Inhale deeply and lengthen your spine.

5. As you exhale, gently twist your torso to the right. Place your left elbow on the outside of your right knee, using it as leverage to deepen the twist. Your right hand can rest behind you for support.

6. You should feel a gentle stretch in your lower back on the left side. This is the quadratus lumborum muscle.

7. Hold this stretch for 15-30 seconds while maintaining deep and controlled breathing.

8. Inhale as you slowly release the twist and return to the center.

9. Repeat the same sequence on the other side to target the right quadratus lumborum muscle.

Supine Quadratus Lumborum Stretch:

1. Lie on your back with your legs extended.

2. Bend your knees and bring them toward your chest.

3. Cross your right ankle over your left thigh, just above your knee.

4. Clasp your hands behind your left thigh.

5. Gently pull your left knee toward your chest to feel the stretch in your lower back on the right side, specifically in the right quadratus lumborum muscle.

6. Hold this stretch for 15-30 seconds.

7. Inhale deeply and release your leg.

8. Repeat the same sequence on the other side to target the left quadratus lumborum muscle.

You may greatly improve the flexibility and comfort of your lower back by integrating these seated and supine quadratus lumborum stretches into your daily routine. Remember to focus on deep and regulated breathing while you perform these stretches to improve relaxation and muscle release.

These stretches can be done at any time of day that is convenient for you. You might do them in the morning to start your day with a relaxed lower back or in the evening to relieve discomfort and prepare for a comfortable night's sleep.

Gentle Spinal Twists and Stretches on the Floor: Maintaining Spinal Flexibility

Maintaining spinal flexibility is essential for overall mobility and comfort, particularly as we age. Gentle spinal twists and stretches on the floor are effective ways to target the muscles and connective tissues that run along your spine. These stretches can help relieve pain, increase range of motion, and promote relaxation in your back and core.

Understanding the Importance of Spinal Flexibility:

The spine, also known as the vertebral column, is an important component in your body that supports and protects your spinal cord while allowing you to move freely. Bending, reaching, and twisting are all movements that require a flexible spine. However, age, prolonged sitting, and a sedentary lifestyle can lead to decreased spinal flexibility, potentially causing discomfort, limited range of motion, and an increased risk of back pain.

How to Perform Gentle Spinal Twists and Stretches:

Let's explore how to perform gentle spinal twists and stretches effectively:

Supine Spinal Twist:

1. Lie on your back with your legs extended.

2. Bend your knees and bring them toward your chest.

3. Extend your arms out to the sides, forming a "T" shape.

4. Inhale deeply and, as you exhale, gently lower both knees to one side, keeping your shoulders grounded on the floor.

5. You should feel a gentle twist in your spine. This targets the muscles along the sides of your spine.

6. Hold the stretch for 15-30 seconds while maintaining deep and controlled breathing.

7. Inhale as you return your knees to the center.

8. Repeat the same sequence by twisting your knees to the opposite side.

Cat-Cow Stretch:

1. Begin on your hands and knees in a tabletop position.

2. Inhale deeply and arch your back, lifting your head and tailbone toward the ceiling. This is the "cow" position.

3. Exhale and round your back, tucking your chin and tailbone. This is the "cat" position.

4. Repeat this movement, flowing between cat and cow, for 30 seconds.

Child's Pose:

1. Kneel on the floor with your big toes touching and knees spread apart.

2. Sit back on your heels and stretch your arms forward on the floor.

3. Lower your chest toward the floor while keeping your arms extended.

4. Hold this stretch for 30 seconds.

You can improve your spine's flexibility and comfort by including these simple spinal twists and stretches into your everyday routine. Remember to focus on deep and regulated breathing while you complete these stretches to improve relaxation and muscle release.

These stretches can be done at any time of day that is convenient for you. You might practice them in the morning to gently awaken your spine or in the evening to relax your back and prepare for a comfortable night's sleep.

Chapter 7

Improving Balance and Stability

Balance and stability are fundamental to maintaining independence and preventing falls, especially as we age. In this chapter, we'll explore various exercises and movements that focus on enhancing your balance and stability. These activities are designed to help you feel more confident in your daily life and reduce the risk of falls.

Standing on One Leg for Balance: Finding Your Center

Standing on one leg may appear to be a simple exercise, but it is a potent one for improving balance, stability, and even mental focus. While it is frequently overlooked, the ability to stand on one leg is essential for many daily activities, including putting on pants, reaching for objects on high shelves, and stepping over obstacles. This activity becomes increasingly important as we age in order to preserve independence and lessen the chance of falling. In this section, we'll go over the significance of this exercise, its advantages, and variants, and how to incorporate it into your regular routine.

Importance of Standing on One Leg:

Standing on one leg is a good indicator of one's overall balance and stability. Standing on one leg engages several muscle groups, including those in your core, hips, and ankles. These muscles collaborate to keep you upright and stable. As you continue to do this, you will develop these muscles, which will contribute to better balance and general stability.

Balance is an important part of preserving independence because it has a direct impact on your daily life. Simple acts such as getting out of a chair, stepping onto a curb, or walking over uneven surfaces all necessitate a solid sense of balance. You can perform these activities with greater confidence and comfort if you have better balance, which reduces the possibility of accidents or injuries.

Benefits of Standing on One Leg:

Practicing standing on one leg offers numerous benefits for seniors:

1. **Improved Balance**: The primary benefit is, of course, improved balance. By challenging your body to balance on one leg, you train your muscles and central nervous system to work together more efficiently, enhancing your ability to maintain equilibrium.

2. **Strengthened Leg Muscles**: Standing on one leg targets and strengthens the muscles in your supporting leg. This includes the quadriceps, hamstrings, and calf muscles, which are essential for maintaining stability and preventing falls.

3. **Enhanced Core Strength**: Balancing on one leg also engages your core muscles. A strong core provides

better support for your spine, reduces the risk of lower back pain, and aids in maintaining an upright posture.

4. **Better Proprioception**: Proprioception is your body's sense of where it is in space. Practicing balance exercises enhances your proprioception, which is valuable for preventing falls and maintaining overall mobility.

5. **Mental Focus**: Balance exercises demand mental concentration. Practicing standing on one leg can sharpen your cognitive abilities and increase mindfulness, which is beneficial for overall mental well-being.

How to Stand on One Leg:

To practice standing on one leg effectively, follow these steps:

Find Your Starting Position: Begin by standing up straight with your feet hip-width apart. Ensure you're in a safe and clutter-free space.

Engage Your Core: Activate your core muscles by gently pulling your navel toward your spine. This action stabilizes your posture.

Lift One Leg: Slowly raise one foot off the ground. You can start with your dominant or non-dominant leg; the choice is yours. Begin by bending your knee at a 90-degree angle.

Find a Focal Point: Choose a point in front of you to focus on. This will help you maintain your balance by fixing your gaze on a single spot.

Hold the Position: Attempt to stand on one leg for 10-15 seconds. If this feels challenging, start with a shorter duration and work your way up gradually. Don't be discouraged by initial wobbling; it's a sign that your body is adjusting and growing stronger.

Switch Sides: Carefully lower your raised leg and shift your weight to the other leg. Repeat the exercise with your other leg. Be mindful of the transition to avoid any sudden movements.

Challenge Yourself: Once you feel comfortable standing on one leg with your eyes open, consider trying it with your eyes closed. This adds an extra layer of complexity as it removes the visual sense, forcing your muscles and proprioception to work even harder.

Variations and Progressions:

As you become more proficient at standing on one leg, you can introduce variations and progressions to challenge yourself further and enhance your balance:

1. **Leg Swings**: While standing on one leg, gently swing your raised leg forward and backward or side to side. This dynamic movement adds a layer of complexity to the exercise.

2. **Arm Movements**: Extend your arms to the sides or overhead while standing on one leg. This increases the challenge by altering your center of gravity.

3. **Changing Surfaces**: Try standing on a slightly cushioned surface, like a foam pad or a folded yoga mat. This introduces an element of instability, which can benefit balance training.

4. **Tandem Stance**: In the tandem stance, place the heel of your raised foot against the toes of your supporting foot. This narrows your base of support and makes the exercise more challenging.

5. **Dynamic Movements**: Combine standing on one leg with other activities, such as arm reaches, small knee bends, or head turns. These dynamic movements mimic real-life situations that require a combination of balance and coordination.

Incorporating Standing on One Leg into Your Daily Routine:

Standing on one leg is an exercise that can be seamlessly integrated into your daily routine. Here are some tips to help you make it a consistent part of your life:

1. **Start Your Day:** Begin your day with a few minutes of standing on one leg while you brush your teeth or wait for your morning coffee to brew.

2. **TV Time:** Use the time when you're watching TV to practice balance exercises. During commercial breaks or at the end of an episode, stand on one leg for a minute or two.

3. **Kitchen Moments:** While you're waiting for water to boil or your oven to preheat, practice your balance by standing on one leg.

4. **Outdoor Balance:** If you have access to a safe outdoor space, take your balance practice outside. The fresh air and change of scenery can enhance your experience.

5. **Accountability Partner:** If you have a friend or family member who's also interested in balance exercises, consider doing it together. Accountability partners can help you stay motivated.

6. **Set a Timer:** Use a timer or smartphone app to track your progress. Gradually increase the duration as you become more comfortable.

Remember that consistency is essential. The more you practice standing on one leg, the better your balance and stability will be. Be patient with yourself as well. Although progress is slow, every second spent on one leg is a step toward improving your well-being and independence. So, stand tall, find your center, and enjoy the many advantages of this seemingly easy yet highly beneficial exercise.

Toe Taps and Heel Raises for Stability: Strengthening Your Lower Extremities

Toe taps and heel raises are simple but effective exercises for improving lower-extremity stability and strength, particularly in the ankles and calves. These exercises are not only important for keeping balance but also for preventing falls because strong ankles and calves help to stabilize your body during varied motions. In this section, we'll look at the significance of toe taps and heel rises, how to do them correctly, the benefits of doing them, and how to incorporate them into your daily routine.

Importance of Toe Taps and Heel Raises:

The ankles and calves are important in maintaining balance and stability. They aid in the stabilization of your body, whether standing, walking, or even sprinting. Toe taps and heel raises are exercises that especially target and develop the muscles in these areas.

Fall prevention begins with strengthening your ankles and calves. Falls are frequently caused by instability in the lower extremities. These muscles can better support your weight and help you maintain balance even in difficult situations if they are strong and well-conditioned.

How to Perform Toe Taps and Heel Raises:

Let's break down how to perform these two exercises correctly:

Toe Taps:

1. Begin by finding a sturdy surface to hold onto for support, such as the back of a chair, a countertop, or a wall.

2. Stand tall with your feet hip-width apart.

3. Keep your heels on the ground while lifting your toes off the ground in a controlled manner.

4. Gently tap your toes forward and then return them to the ground.

5. Perform 10-15 toe taps, making sure to maintain your balance throughout the exercise.

Heel Raises:

1. Similar to toe taps, begin by standing tall with your feet hip-width apart.

2. This time, lift your heels off the ground, rising onto your toes.

3. Hold this position for a moment to feel the stretch in your calf muscles.

4. Lower your heels back to the ground.

5. Perform 10-15 heel raises, focusing on your balance and control.

Safety Tip: If you feel unsteady, it's perfectly fine to hold onto your support surface, like the back of a chair, while performing these exercises. As your balance and strength improve, you can gradually reduce the support you rely on.

Variations and Progressions:

As you become more confident with toe taps and heel raises, you can introduce variations to challenge yourself and enhance your stability and strength:

1. Single-Leg Variations: Perform toe taps and heel raises while standing on one leg. This adds an extra layer of complexity and further strengthens the supporting leg.

2. Eyes-Closed Challenge: Once you feel comfortable with the exercises, try doing them with your eyes closed. This increases the difficulty as it removes the visual sense, forcing your body to rely more on proprioception — the sense that allows you to know where your body is in space.

3. Incorporate Balance Boards: If you have access to balance boards or wobble boards, these can be excellent tools to challenge your balance further while doing toe taps and heel raises.

Incorporating Toe Taps and Heel Raises into Your Daily Routine:

Making these exercises a part of your daily life doesn't have to be complicated. Here are some practical tips to help you integrate toe taps and heel raises into your routine:

1. **Morning Routine:** Incorporate toe taps and heel raises into your morning routine. While waiting for your coffee to brew or your tea to steep, you can perform these exercises.

2. **TV Time:** Utilize the time when you're watching TV to practice toe taps and heel raises. During commercial breaks or at the end of an episode, perform a few sets.

3. **Kitchen Activities:** Whether you're waiting for water to boil or your oven to preheat, these are great moments to focus on balance exercises.

4. **Outdoor Practice:** If you have access to a safe outdoor space, consider taking your exercises outside. The change of scenery and fresh air can make your practice more enjoyable.

5. **Accountability:** If you have a friend or family member who's also interested in these exercises, you can do them together. Accountability partners can help keep you motivated.

6. **Set Goals:** Set specific goals for the number of toe taps and heel raises you want to achieve each day. Gradually increase the repetitions as you become more comfortable.

Consistency is essential. The more frequently you perform toe taps and heel raises, the higher the benefits you'll enjoy in terms of enhanced lower-extremity stability and strength. These simple but effective exercises can significantly improve your ability to maintain balance, lowering your chance of falling and allowing you to live a more confident and independent life. So, let us begin each day with stronger ankles and calves, ready to face the world with grace and steadiness.

Tai Chi-Inspired Movements for Balance and Coordination: The Flowing Path to Stability

Tai Chi, commonly referred to as "meditation in motion," is a centuries-old Chinese practice that combines soft, flowing motions with deep breathing and mental concentration. While it is well-known for its meditative and stress-relieving benefits, it is also an excellent exercise for improving balance, coordination, and overall stability, making it particularly good for seniors. This section will go into the realm of Tai Chi-inspired motions, their importance, how to do them, their benefits, and how to incorporate this beautiful practice into your daily life.

Importance of Tai Chi-Inspired Movements:

Tai Chi is distinguished by its slow, deliberate movements that flow smoothly from one to the next. Balance, flexibility, strength, and mental attention are all required for these motions. Traditional Chinese medicine and philosophy, which emphasize the need of harmony and balance in all aspects of life, including physical health, are at the basis of the practice.

Balance and coordination are critical for seniors in their daily activities. Maintaining these abilities lowers the likelihood of falls and injury. Tai Chi-inspired motions promote a sense of well-being and tranquility by engaging both the body and mind.

How to Perform Tai Chi-Inspired Movements:

Learning Tai Chi movements may seem daunting at first, but they are designed to be accessible to people of all ages and fitness levels. Here's a basic introduction to getting started:

1. **Find a Quiet Space:** Start by finding a quiet, clutter-free space where you can move without distractions. It's preferable to practice on a non-slip surface or use a non-slip mat.

2. **Wear Comfortable Clothing:** Wear loose, comfortable clothing that allows you to move freely. Tai Chi is typically practiced barefoot or in soft, flat shoes.

3. **Warm-Up:** Begin with a gentle warm-up to prepare your body for movement. This can include light stretching or deep breathing exercises.

4. **Learn Basic Movements:** Tai Chi consists of a series of choreographed movements or forms. Start with the basic movements, such as "Grasp the Sparrow's Tail" or

"Waving Hands Like Clouds." These movements are designed to be performed slowly and gracefully.

5. **Focus on Breathing:** Pay close attention to your breathing. In Tai Chi, the breath should be slow, deep, and coordinated with your movements. As you move, inhale and exhale in a controlled manner.

6. **Maintain Good Posture:** Keep an upright posture with a straight back and relaxed shoulders. Your head should be held as if suspended from above, and your movements should flow from your core.

7. **Practice Regularly:** Consistency is key in Tai Chi. It's better to practice for a short period each day than for a long time once in a while. This helps build muscle memory and improve balance and coordination.

Advantages of Tai Chi-Inspired Movements:

The benefits of Tai Chi-inspired movements are numerous and far-reaching, especially for seniors:

1. **Enhanced Balance:** Tai Chi movements challenge your balance and coordination, helping to reduce the risk of falls.

2. **Improved Flexibility:** The flowing, slow movements gently stretch and strengthen muscles and joints, promoting flexibility.

3. **Mental Focus:** Tai Chi requires mental concentration, which can help improve cognitive function and reduce stress.

4. **Stress Reduction:** The mindful and meditative nature of Tai Chi is known to reduce stress and improve overall mental well-being.

5. **Strength and Endurance:** Despite its gentle appearance, Tai Chi can help build strength and muscular endurance, particularly in the legs and core.

6. **Better Posture:** Practicing good posture is fundamental to Tai Chi, and over time, it can translate into improved posture in daily life.

Incorporating Tai Chi-Inspired Movements into Your Daily Routine:

Integrating Tai Chi-inspired movements into your daily life is a journey of mindfulness and well-being. Here are some tips to make this graceful practice a part of your routine:

1. **Short Sessions:** Begin with short sessions, aiming for just 10-15 minutes a day. As you become more comfortable, gradually increase the duration.

2. **Morning Ritual:** Make Tai Chi-inspired movements a part of your morning ritual. It's a fantastic way to start your day with balance and calm.

3. **Lunchtime Break:** If you have a break during the day, consider dedicating a few minutes to your practice. It can help refresh your mind and energize your body.

4. **Evening Wind-Down:** Use Tai Chi as a way to wind down in the evening. It can help you relax, reduce stress, and prepare for a peaceful night's sleep.

5. **Community Classes:** Many communities offer Tai Chi classes. Joining a class can provide a sense of community and motivation to keep up with your practice.

6. **Online Resources:** If in-person classes aren't accessible, many online resources, videos, and tutorials can guide you through Tai Chi movements.

Incorporating Tai Chi-inspired movements into your daily life can be a rewarding and transformative experience. As you move gracefully and mindfully through these exercises, you'll enhance your balance and coordination and cultivate a sense of harmony and well-being in your daily life. The path to stability and tranquility starts with a single step, or in the case of Tai Chi, a flowing and graceful movement.

Chapter 8

Incorporating Props for

Enhanced Flexibility

We frequently ignore the crucial partners that come in the form of props in our quest to improve flexibility and mobility. These items, whether a basic yoga strap, a foam roller, or a sturdy chair, can take our flexibility exercise to the next level. In this section, we'll look at how to use props to improve your flexibility, get a deeper stretch, and increase general well-being.

Using a Yoga Strap or Towel for Assisted Stretches

Flexibility is frequently seen as the key to preserving your body's youthful vigor and avoiding stiffness and discomfort as you age. While it may be tempting to believe that increasing flexibility necessitates sophisticated exercises or hours of dedicated training, the truth is that basic things such as a yoga strap or towel can make a major difference. This section will go into the world of assisted stretches, how these unassuming instruments may help you unlock your inner flexibility, and how to incorporate them into your everyday routine properly.

The Magic of Assisted Stretches:

Assisted stretches are a simple yet effective approach for increasing flexibility. They entail stretching with a yoga strap or a towel to support your body. These props function as an extension of your arms, helping you to reach farther, hold stretches for longer periods of time, and progressively enhance your range of motion. This is especially useful for seniors and anyone trying to improve their flexibility.

How to Use a Yoga Strap or Towel:

Using a yoga strap or towel for assisted stretches is accessible and can be done at your own pace. Here's a step-by-step guide:

1. **Choose the Right Strap or Towel:** Start by selecting a yoga strap or towel that suits your needs. Most yoga straps are about 6 feet long, and towels should be long enough to provide sufficient support.

2. **Prepare for Your Stretch:** Find a quiet and clutter-free space to perform your stretches. Consider using a non-slip mat for extra stability, especially if you're on a hard surface.

3. **Wrap the Strap or Towel:** Sit down and extend your legs in front of you. Wrap the strap or towel around the sole of one foot, holding one end in each hand. Position your hands closer or further apart along the strap to create the right level of tension for your stretch.

4. **Perform the Stretch:** Gently pull on the strap or towel with your hands to guide your foot closer to your body. This action deepens the stretch in your hamstrings, calves, or other targeted muscle groups. It's important to remember that you should not force the stretch – it should be a gentle and gradual progression. Hold the

stretch for 15-30 seconds while breathing deeply and evenly.

5. **Switch Sides:** After completing the stretch on one side, switch to the other and repeat the process.

Benefits of Using a Yoga Strap or Towel:

The advantages of using a yoga strap or towel for assisted stretches are numerous and can contribute to your overall well-being:

1. **Enhanced Flexibility:** By supporting your stretches, these props allow you to perform them more deeply and effectively. This can accelerate your progress in terms of flexibility and range of motion.

2. **Reduced Risk of Injury:** Assisted stretches are gentle on your muscles and joints, minimizing the risk of overstretching or straining. This can be especially crucial for individuals with mobility concerns or new to stretching exercises.

3. **Increased Range of Motion:** Regular use of a strap or towel can help you gradually expand your range of motion, making everyday movements easier and more comfortable.

4. **Relaxation and Stress Reduction:** Deep stretches with a strap or towel can promote relaxation, reduce muscle tension, and help alleviate stress. The meditative aspect of stretching can also provide mental and emotional benefits.

Tips for Using a Yoga Strap or Towel:

To make the most of assisted stretches, consider these practical tips:

1. **Stay Relaxed:** When using a strap or towel, relaxing into the stretch is essential rather than forcing it. Listen to your body and avoid pushing yourself too far or too quickly.

2. **Breathe Mindfully:** Focus on your breath during the stretch. Inhale deeply and exhale slowly, allowing your breath to guide your body deeper into the stretch and enhance relaxation.

3. **Consistency is Key:** Incorporate assisted stretches into your daily routine. Consistency is more important than the duration of a single stretch session, as it helps your body adapt and improve over time.

Incorporating Assisted Stretches into Your Daily Routine:

To make assisted stretches a consistent part of your daily routine, consider the following suggestions:

1. **Morning Ritual:** Start your day with a few minutes of assisted stretches using your strap or towel. This can help wake up your muscles, increase circulation, and promote flexibility from the get-go.

2. **Short Breaks:** Throughout your day, whether at work or during a leisure activity, take short breaks to do a couple of assisted stretches. These can help relieve tension and reenergize your body and mind.

3. **Evening Wind-Down:** Wind down in the evening by using your strap or towel for gentle stretches. This can assist in relaxation, stress reduction, and preparing your body for a restful night's sleep.

4. **Community Classes:** If available, consider joining community yoga or flexibility classes. These sessions often provide guidance on how to effectively use props and offer a sense of community and motivation to continue your practice.

Stretching using a yoga strap or towel might be a game changer on your path to greater flexibility. These simple tools allow you to reach further, stretch deeper, and progressively improve your flexibility while reducing your chance of injury. You may reap the benefits of a more flexible and mobile body by incorporating assisted stretches into your daily routine, enhancing your overall health and well-being.

Incorporating a Foam Roller for Myofascial Release and Stretching

The foam roller emerges as a fascinating instrument that can work wonders for your muscles and overall well-being in the quest for better flexibility and mobility. This cylindrical piece of dense foam, which is often overlooked, has garnered recognition for its effectiveness in myofascial release, stretching, and flexibility enhancement. In this section, we'll delve into the realm of foam rolling, learning how it works, its benefits, and how to include it into your daily routine.

Understanding Myofascial Release:

Myofascial release is a therapy that focuses on the fascia, which is a connective tissue that surrounds and supports the body's muscles, bones, and organs. Tight or restricted fascia can cause discomfort, limited flexibility, and even pain. Myofascial release is a technique that uses pressure to remove fascial tension, allowing muscles to move more easily.

How Foam Rolling Works:

A foam roller, usually made of high-density foam, is your entry point into myofascial release. It uses your body weight to apply pressure to various parts of your body, relieving tension, increasing flexibility, and improving general mobility. This self-massage effect aids in releasing knots, increases blood flow, and reduces muscle tension.

Using a Foam Roller:

Let's break down how to effectively use a foam roller in your flexibility and mobility routine:

1. **Choose the Right Foam Roller**: Foam rollers come in various densities, from soft to firm. If you're a beginner or new to foam rolling, start with a softer roller. As you become accustomed to the practice, you can transition to firmer options for deeper pressure.

2. **Find a Comfortable Space**: Select a comfortable, flat surface to roll on. A yoga mat or a carpet can provide cushioning and support.

3. Start Slow: Initiate the practice with gentle pressure. Position the foam roller under the muscle group you wish to work on.

4. **Apply Pressure**: With the foam roller in place, gently roll back and forth over the targeted muscle area. If you encounter a particularly tight or tender spot, pause and hold the pressure on that point for about 20-30 seconds. This allows the muscles to release and relax.

5. **Breathe Mindfully**: Throughout the process, maintain mindful and deep breathing. This practice helps you relax and promotes the release of tension in the muscles.

6. **Cover Different Areas**: Continue rolling, focusing on various muscle groups, and pay attention to areas that may feel tight or need relief.

Benefits of Foam Rolling:

The use of a foam roller in your flexibility routine offers a multitude of benefits that contribute to your overall well-being:

1. Improved Flexibility: Regular foam rolling aids in the release of tight fascia, which may restrict movement. This can lead to improved flexibility and range of motion.

2. Reduced Muscle Soreness: Foam rolling is particularly beneficial after a workout. It helps reduce muscle soreness and facilitates faster recovery.

3. Enhanced Circulation: The pressure applied during foam rolling increases blood flow to the muscles, contributing to the healing process and promoting overall health.

4. Injury Prevention: By releasing muscle tension and maintaining flexibility, foam rolling can help prevent injuries related to tight muscles and restricted movement.

5. Relaxation and Stress Reduction: Foam rolling can be a relaxing and meditative practice to reduce stress and improve emotional well-being.

Incorporating Foam Rolling into Your Daily Routine:

To effectively integrate foam rolling into your daily life and reap the benefits it offers, consider the following suggestions:

1. **Pre-Workout Routine:** Spend a few minutes foam rolling before starting your workout. This prepares your muscles and joints for exercise, allowing for better performance and reducing the risk of injury.

2. **Post-Workout Recovery:** After exercising, use the foam roller to reduce muscle soreness and expedite your recovery process.

3. **Evening Wind-Down:** Incorporate foam rolling into your evening routine to relax and release tension from the day, promoting a sense of calm and well-being.

4. **Target Specific Areas:** Focus on areas that feel tight or tense, such as the calves, quadriceps, hamstrings, and the back. Tailor your foam rolling routine to address your specific needs.

Foam rolling is a versatile and effective technique for improving flexibility, reducing muscle tension, and promoting overall well-being. By incorporating this exercise into your daily routine on a regular basis, you can see a significant improvement in your flexibility, mobility, and overall quality of life. The benefits of foam rolling are available to everyone who is prepared to explore its potential.

Chair Yoga with Props for Additional Support and Flexibility

Chair yoga is a type of yoga that modifies the practice for people with different levels of mobility, making it accessible to everyone. This modified type of yoga uses a chair as a prop to provide additional support, stability, and flexibility for those who may find regular yoga difficult due to physical constraints. In this section, we'll examine the world of chair yoga, its numerous benefits, and how integrating props can improve your practice by providing more flexibility and balance.

The Allure of Chair Yoga:

Chair yoga is intended to make yoga more accessible by allowing those with various physical impairments to enjoy the numerous benefits of yoga without having to get down on the floor. The chair provides stability and support, making it a safer option for people who are prone to falling or have problems balancing during traditional yoga sessions.

Advantages of Chair Yoga:

1. **Enhanced Flexibility**: Chair yoga encourages gentle stretching and flexibility, which can be especially

beneficial for seniors or individuals with limited mobility. The use of props like straps and blocks can further enhance these stretches.

2. **Improved Balance:** The chair's support allows participants to work on balance in a safe and controlled environment. By gradually incorporating balance-focused poses and movements, individuals can strengthen their core and improve overall stability.

3. **Reduced Risk of Injury:** Chair yoga minimizes the risk of injury associated with traditional yoga, making it suitable for those with physical limitations or those recovering from injuries.

4. **Stress Reduction:** Chair yoga doesn't skimp on the mental and emotional benefits of traditional yoga. The mindfulness and relaxation aspects remain integral to the practice, helping to alleviate stress and improve emotional well-being.

Utilizing Props in Chair Yoga:

Props are a significant component of chair yoga, enhancing your practice and offering additional support. Here are some props commonly used in chair yoga:

1. **Yoga Straps:** Straps can help you achieve a deeper stretch, particularly in seated or standing poses.

2. **Blocks**: Blocks are excellent for modifying poses and making them more accessible. They provide extra support for hands or feet, helping you maintain proper alignment.

3. **Cushions and Bolsters**: These props can provide additional comfort during seated poses, offering extra cushioning and support.

4. **Blankets**: Blankets are often used for added warmth and comfort, particularly during relaxation and meditation exercises.

5. **Chairs**: The chair itself is a primary prop in chair yoga. It provides stability and support during standing poses, balance exercises, and more.

How to Incorporate Props into Chair Yoga:

Incorporating props into chair yoga is both accessible and effective. Here's how to do it:

1. **Choose the Right Props**: Select the props that align with your specific needs and the type of chair yoga you're practicing. These props can be easily found in yoga and fitness stores or online.

2. **Prop Placement:** Follow the guidance of your chair yoga instructor on how to use props effectively. They can assist you in finding the best placement for added support or deeper stretches.

3. **Prioritize Safety**: When using props, always prioritize safety. Ensure that props are secure and won't compromise your balance or stability.

4. **Listen to Your Body**: As with any yoga practice, listening to your body is crucial. If a particular prop doesn't work for you or feels uncomfortable, feel free to make adjustments or ask for guidance from your instructor.

Incorporating Chair Yoga with Props into Your Daily Routine:

To make chair yoga with props a consistent part of your daily routine, consider the following suggestions:

1. Morning Practice: Start your day with a chair yoga session that includes the use of props. This can help you feel energized, flexible, and balanced throughout the day.

2. Short Breaks: Incorporate short chair yoga breaks into your daily routine. For instance, take a few minutes to do chair yoga stretches and deep breathing exercises during work breaks or while watching TV.

3. Evening Relaxation: Use chair yoga with props to wind down in the evening. This can help you relax, reduce stress, and prepare for a peaceful night's sleep.

4. Community Classes: If available, consider joining chair yoga classes in your community. These classes often provide access to props and expert guidance.

Chair yoga with props is a very adaptive and accessible practice that delivers yoga benefits to various people. By incorporating this activity into your daily life, you can enhance your flexibility, balance, and overall well-being. It provides a path to improved mobility and a greater connection between your body and mind, ultimately improving the quality of your life. So, pick a comfortable chair, gather your props, and let chair yoga guide you to greater flexibility and stability.

Chapter 9

Incorporating Mindfulness and

Breathing

In our ongoing journey to boost flexibility, there's a powerful yet often overlooked ally—mindfulness, coupled with mindful breathing techniques. This combination can amplify your stretching and mobility exercises, helping you reach new heights of flexibility and well-being. In this chapter, we'll explore the profound effects of mindfulness and breath awareness on your flexibility journey, delve into the intricacies of combining relaxation and stretching, and understand how focused awareness of your muscles can transform your results.

Mindful Breathing Techniques During Stretching and Mobility Exercises

Incorporating mindful breathing into your stretching and mobility exercises can be a life-changing experience, enriching your path to greater flexibility and general well-being. Conscious breathing greatly affects your physical and mental state, leading you through each stretch and allowing you to achieve new levels of flexibility. We'll delve deeper into the world of mindful breathing in this expanded exploration, learning its fundamentals, how it impacts your body and practical strategies for adopting it into your everyday routine.

The Mind-Body Connection:

Before going into the mechanics of mindful breathing during stretching and mobility exercises, it's critical to understand the mind-body relationship. Our mental and physical states are inextricably linked; they influence and respond to one another in a dynamic dance of sensations, emotions, and experiences. This connection is the basis for mindfulness, a practice that teaches us to be fully present in the moment without judgment or distraction.

Mindful Breathing Defined:

Mindful breathing is an essential component of mindfulness. It entails paying close attention to your breath (inhales and exhales) without seeking to control or manage it. Instead, you become a neutral spectator, curiously and nonjudgmentally watching your breath. When combined with stretching and mobility exercises, mindful breathing can serve as a reliable guide.

The Impact of Mindful Breathing on Flexibility:

The connection between mindful breathing and flexibility is a symbiotic one. As you engage in your stretches with deliberate breath awareness, you invite several profound benefits:

1. Enhancing Flexibility and Range of Motion:

Consider each breath as an invitation to your body to go deeper into your stretches. There is a gentle release of tension when you exhale, enabling your muscles to relax and your body to sink deeper into the stretch. This regular inhaling and exhaling exercise can lead to an increased range of motion over time.

2. Stress Reduction and Relaxation:

Mindful breathing has the ability to alleviate tension and induce relaxation by itself. Focusing on your breath activates your parasympathetic nerve system, sometimes called the "rest and digest" system. This calm state helps your stretching practice, allowing your muscles to relax more deeply.

3. Heightened Mind-Body Awareness:

Mindful breathing helps you become more aware of your body. Stretching and breathing increase your awareness of physiological feelings and feedback. This sensory awareness helps you identify areas of tension or discomfort and modify your activities to relieve them.

4. Guided Movements:

Your breath acts as an internal guidance for your motions. You may ensure that each move is smooth and safe by synchronizing your stretches with your breath. Your breath acts as a conduit between your conscious intentions and physical reality, allowing you to move through your stretching practice easily.

How to Practice Mindful Breathing During Stretching and Mobility Exercises:

1. **Prepare and Center**: Before you embark on your stretching journey, take a moment to prepare. Find a quiet and comfortable space, either sitting or standing, and close your eyes. Let your awareness settle into the present moment.

2. **Connect with Your Breath**: Transition your focus to your breath. Begin to observe each inhalation and

exhalation without trying to manipulate them in any way. This initial step sets the stage for mindfulness.

3. **Synchronize Your Movements**: As you stretch, consciously align them with your breath. As you inhale, prepare for the stretch ahead. As you exhale, gracefully surrender to the movement, allowing your muscles to relax and lengthen.

4. **Release with Exhalation**: Pay close attention to your exhalations. They provide a natural opportunity to release tension. Visualize your muscles elongating and relaxing as you breathe out, allowing the stretch to become deeper and more effective.

5. **Stay Present:** Throughout your flexibility exercises, maintain a vigilant presence with your breath. If your mind starts to wander, gently bring your attention to your breath and the sensations within your body.

Each movement becomes an intentional and completely present experience when mindful breathing is incorporated into your stretching and mobility exercises. This method not only promotes better flexibility but also cultivates a profound mind-body connection, which can lead to improved physical performance. Your breath becomes a meditative companion while you practice, accompanying you on the path to greater flexibility and well-being.

Cultivating Mindful Breathing in Your Daily Life:

To integrate mindful breathing into your daily life, consider these practices:

1. **Morning Mindfulness**: Begin your day with a few moments of mindful breathing. Sit quietly, close your eyes, and focus on your breath. Let this practice set a positive tone for the day.

2. **Mindful Meals**: During your meals, devote your full attention to the flavors, textures, and smells of your food. This not only enhances awareness but also aids in digestion.

3. **Mindful Breaks**: Throughout your day, take short, mindful breaks. Step away from your tasks, breathe deeply, and observe the present moment. This can refresh your mind and reduce stress.

4. **Evening Wind-Down**: Before bedtime, engage in mindful breathing or body scan exercises to relax and prepare for restful sleep.

5. **Mindful Stretching**: Incorporate mindful breathing and focused awareness into your stretching and mobility routine, as discussed in this chapter.

You can create a better feeling of presence, reduce stress, and improve your general well-being by gradually incorporating mindfulness and breath awareness into your daily life. Integrating these activities can be a game changer for your flexibility journey, improving both your physical skills and your inner peace. Combined with relaxation, stretching, and mindfulness, they form a perfect synergy that promotes deep flexibility and a profound connection between body and mind.

Focused Awareness on Muscles Being Stretched for Better Results

Improving your flexibility and mobility requires both physical and mental effort. A great approach for deepening your connection between body and mind during stretching and mobility exercises is focused awareness of the muscles being stretched. In this section, we will go into the relevance of the muscle-mind connection, how it affects stretching results, and practical strategies to incorporate it into your everyday routine.

Understanding the Muscle-Mind Connection:

The muscle-mind connection, also called the mind-muscle connection, is a key concept in physical health and exercise. It requires paying attention to certain muscle groups while performing various physical exercises. Rather than just going through the motions, this practice consciously directs your attention to the muscles employed during a certain movement or exercise.

This increased awareness allows you to connect with your body more intimately. It entails sensing and understanding individual muscles' tension, contraction, and release as they strive to accomplish a specific task. You build a stronger feeling of physical awareness by actively engaging in the muscle-mind connection, allowing you to perform precise and intentional motions.

This practice improves the efficacy of your workouts and lowers your chance of injury by ensuring that your muscles are appropriately engaged and aligned throughout the activity. Finally, the muscle-mind link lets you improve your physical performance and get more out of your workout routines.

The Impact of Muscle-Mind Connection on Flexibility:

Creating a strong muscle-mind connection during your stretching and mobility exercises can lead to several profound benefits:

1. Enhanced Flexibility and Range of Motion:

By concentrating your attention on the muscles you're stretching, you can help them relax and release tension more effectively. This can lead to a deeper and more productive stretch, which can improve your general flexibility and range of motion over time.

2. Improved Muscle Control:

The muscle-mind connection allows you to become more aware of your body. You develop more control over certain muscle groups, which is especially useful in exercises that target specific portions of your body, such as hip flexors or hamstrings.

3. Enhanced Safety:

Being aware of your muscles' responses to stretching can help you avoid overstretching, which can lead to injury. You may be more exact in your movements with a strong muscle-mind connection, ensuring your stretches are both effective and safe.

4. Mindful Progression:

You can track your progress more effectively by being in tune with your muscles. You'll notice when your muscles become more pliable and when you can achieve a deeper stretch, allowing you to tailor your exercises to your evolving needs.

Practical Techniques for Muscle-Mind Connection:

1. **Start with Body Scan**: Before you begin your stretching routine, take a moment to perform a mental body scan. Close your eyes and mentally explore your body, paying attention to areas that may feel tense or tight. This sets the stage for focused awareness.

2. **Identify Targeted Muscles**: During each stretch, identify the specific muscle or muscle group you're targeting. For example, if you're performing a hamstring stretch, consciously focus on your hamstring muscles.

3. **Visualize Muscle Engagement**: As you initiate the stretch, visualize the muscle or muscles elongating and relaxing. Imagine them softening and yielding to the stretch. This mental imagery enhances muscle relaxation.

4. **Mindful Breathing**: Combine muscle awareness with mindful breathing. As you breathe, direct your breath

toward the muscle you're stretching. Imagine the breath helping the muscle release tension.

5. **Use Verbal Cues**: Sometimes, using verbal cues can help. Mentally repeat the name of the muscle you're stretching. For instance, if you're stretching your quadriceps, silently say "quadriceps" in your mind as you stretch.

6. **Stay Present**: Throughout your stretching routine, focus on the targeted muscle. If your mind starts to wander, gently bring it back to the sensation in the muscle.

7. **Practice Patience**: Cultivating the muscle-mind connection takes practice. Be patient with yourself and allow your awareness to grow over time.

You may improve your entire experience by incorporating the muscle-mind connection into your stretching and mobility exercises. This method promotes a fundamental connection between your body and mind, increasing flexibility, muscle control, and safety. Your exercises will become more intentional and effective as you practice, allowing you to develop on your journey to greater flexibility and mobility.

Cultivating the Muscle-Mind Connection in Your Daily Life:

To integrate the muscle-mind connection into your daily routine, consider the following practices:

1. **Mindful Walking**: Pay attention to the muscles involved in each step during your daily walk. Focus on the sensation in your legs and feet as they move.

2. **Postural Awareness:** As you sit or stand throughout the day, periodically check in with your posture. Pay attention to the muscles that support your spine and alignment.

3. **Functional Movements**: While performing everyday tasks like lifting objects or bending down, engage the muscle-mind connection. Be aware of the muscles required for the activity.

4. **Mindful Workouts**: If you engage in more vigorous workouts, practice the muscle-mind connection during strength and resistance exercises. Focus on the specific muscle groups being used.

5. **Mindful Relaxation:** Even in moments of rest, maintain some muscle awareness. Relaxation techniques like progressive muscle relaxation can help you become more aware of your muscles and their tension levels.

You will build a more profound sense of body awareness by integrating the muscle-mind connection into your daily life. This enhanced connection between your mind and muscles can result in better posture, more effective movement, and a higher appreciation for your body's potential.

Combining Relaxation and Stretching for Improved Flexibility

While primarily concerned with the physical aspect of stretching, flexibility exercises also provide an ideal opportunity to include relaxation techniques into your daily routine. Combining relaxing and stretching can result in a powerful synergy that promotes deeper flexibility, increased mobility, and a sensation of well-being that spreads throughout your entire body and mind.

The Stress-Flexibility Connection:

The link between stress and flexibility is a significant aspect of understanding the dynamics of our bodies during physical activity, particularly stretching. When stressed, our bodies frequently respond by contracting muscles as a natural protection mechanism. This muscle contraction is a reflexive response designed to defend the body from potential threats. However, in the context of flexibility and stretching, it can impede our ability to attain deep and effective stretches.

Stress can also cause shallow breathing patterns. When we are concerned or stressed, our breathing becomes quick and shallow. This breathing pattern hinders oxygen supply to our muscles, reducing their ability to relax and extend. A lack of appropriate oxygen flow can also increase muscular tension and stiffness, further restricting flexibility.

Understanding the link between stress and flexibility is the first step toward comprehending the importance of integrating relaxation techniques with stretching. We offset the negative effects of stress on our bodies by doing so, allowing us to stretch more deeply, access a larger range of motion, and promote physical and emotional well-being. This integration is critical for creating flexibility as well as emotional equilibrium.

The Benefits of Combining Relaxation and Stretching:

1. Enhanced Flexibility: Relaxation techniques help release muscle tension, allowing for deeper and more effective stretches.

2. Improved Range of Motion: As your muscles relax, you can access a broader range of motion, enhancing your flexibility and mobility.

3. Stress Reduction: Combining relaxation with stretching is an excellent way to reduce stress and promote emotional well-being.

4. Pain Relief: Relaxed muscles are less likely to experience pain or discomfort during stretching exercises.

How to Combine Relaxation and Stretching:

1. **Start with Deep Breathing:** Before you begin your stretching routine, take a few moments for deep breathing. Inhale slowly and deeply through your nose, allowing your abdomen to rise and exhale fully through your mouth. This calms your nervous system and prepares your body for relaxation.

2. **Progressive Muscle Relaxation:** As you stretch, engage in progressive muscle relaxation. While in a stretch, take a moment to tense and then release the muscles you're

working consciously. This technique promotes relaxation within the stretch.

3. **Mindful Awareness:** Throughout your stretching routine, maintain mindful awareness. Focus on the sensations in your body, the stretch itself, and the release of tension. This present-moment focus enhances the relaxation aspect of your routine.

4. **Incorporate Visualization:** Use visualization to enhance the relaxation component. As you stretch, visualize your muscles softening and elongating. This mental imagery can help your muscles relax more deeply.

5. **Combine with Breathing Techniques:** Infuse relaxation exercises with mindful breathing. As you exhale, envision tension and stress leaving your body. As you inhale, invite calm and relaxation in.

6. **End with Savasana:** If your stretching routine is part of a longer yoga practice, end with Savasana (corpse pose). This relaxation posture allows you to absorb the benefits of stretching and relaxation efforts.

7. **Calm Your Mind:** Embrace mental relaxation alongside physical relaxation. Let go of worries and stress as you stretch, allowing your mind to be peaceful and meditative.

Combining relaxation and stretching is a potent tool in your quest for flexibility and mobility. By including relaxation techniques in your stretching regimen, you can improve your physical flexibility and mental well-being. This all-encompassing approach promotes a deep sense of calm and tranquility that transcends beyond your flexibility exercises and into your daily life.

Incorporating Mindfulness and Breath in Your Daily Routine:

To make mindfulness and breath awareness an integral part of your daily life, consider the following:

1. **Morning Mindfulness:** Start your day with a few minutes of mindfulness. Sit quietly, close your eyes, and focus on your breath. Allow this practice to set a positive tone for the day.

2. **Mindful Meals:** During meals, pay full attention to the flavors, textures, and smells of your food. This mindful eating practice not only promotes awareness but also aids in digestion.

3. **Mindful Breaks:** Throughout your day, take short, mindful breaks. Step away from your tasks, breathe deeply, and observe the present moment. This can refresh your mind and reduce stress.

4. **Evening Wind-Down:** Before bed, engage in mindful breathing or body scan exercises to relax and prepare for restful sleep.

5. **Mindful Stretching:** Integrate mindful breathing and focused awareness into your stretching and mobility routine, as discussed in this chapter.

You can create a better feeling of presence, reduce stress, and improve your general well-being by gradually incorporating mindfulness and breath awareness into your daily life. Integrating these activities can be a game changer for your flexibility journey, improving both your physical skills and your inner peace. Combined with relaxation, stretching, and mindfulness, they form a perfect synergy that promotes deep flexibility and a profound connection between body and mind.

Chapter 10

Tracking Progress and Adjusting Routines

This chapter will explore the vital components of tracking your progress and adjusting your flexibility and mobility routines. As your journey towards improved flexibility and mobility is ongoing, so is the need to monitor your achievements, evaluate your strategies, and set new goals to maintain motivation. It's a dynamic process; adapting is key to a lifelong commitment to your well-being.

Keeping a Flexibility and Mobility Journal

Maintaining a flexibility and mobility journal is akin to preserving a personal time capsule, a repository of your physical and mental growth throughout your journey toward enhanced well-being. This journal is more than a simple notebook; it becomes an integral part of your daily routine, holding your experiences, achievements, and insights, as well as your challenges and progress. Let's delve into why keeping a journal is not only a helpful practice but a transformative one.

Documenting Your Journey:

Consider your flexibility and mobility journals to be a dedication diary, a live witness to your unwavering dedication to better health. Each entry becomes a chapter in your particular story of perseverance and growth. These entries are more than just numbers or notes; they capture the soul of your everyday efforts, whether modest successes or huge milestones.

You bring your path to life by writing down your experiences, accomplishments, and obstacles. You bear witness to your everyday commitment to your never-ending pursuit of a healthier, more mobile you. These entries serve as a tribute to your persistent dedication, one that is vividly alive rather than confined to memory. In a world where major successes and milestones are frequently celebrated, your notebook encourages you to appreciate and honor the tiny, gradual stages representing growth's core.

Every page in your journal is a testament to your fortitude, a daily reminder that your path is still underway. Even on days when progress appears miniature, these entries validate your dedication and the significance of each step you take. They serve as a reminder of the importance of even seemingly insignificant everyday accomplishments. Your journal is a dynamic, living document that captures the essence of your dedication and growth, day by day.

Tracking Progress:

Your journal acts as a roadmap for your journey to more flexibility and mobility. It's a fantastic tool for tracking progress, providing you with insights about your development that you may otherwise miss. When you sit down to go through previous entries, you start on a journey through your own history of accomplishments, a vivid reminder of your growth.

Each page exposes the steps you've taken, the obstacles you've overcome, and the milestones you've reached. Even on days when the present appears to be devoid of significant change, you can see how far you've come. This voyage through your notebook is similar to retracing your steps in the sands of your flexibility and mobility excursion.

As you analyze past entries, you'll see patterns and trends in your progress. Perhaps you've noticed that some routines or exercises produce more noticeable effects, or you've recognized specific habits that impede your progress. These revelations can be transformative because they give you the knowledge you need to make informed changes to your routine. Your journal transforms from a log to a teacher, providing insights that alter your journey's direction and help you adjust and refine your approach. This list of accomplishments emphasizes that your journey is distinguished by ongoing forward movement, even if the objective is still in sight.

Celebrating the Small Wins:

The threads of small wins weave the most colorful and intricate patterns in the vast tapestry of your flexibility and mobility journey. Your journal is your devoted space to commemorate these small victories, whether big or small. Recognizing these modest triumphs is not only a source of joy; it is also a critical component of maintaining consistent drive.

Your journal acts as a mirror, reflecting the beauty of each small win back to you. It's a space where you may take a moment to appreciate the significance of your everyday efforts, no matter how minor they appear. Every stretch a little deeper, every day a bit more devoted - these small wins form the foundation of your path and deserve to be celebrated.

The act of documenting and appreciating your small accomplishments has a significant impact on your motivation. It's a constant source of motivation that supports the idea that you're on the correct track. This awareness inspires you not just to pursue large goals, but also to recognize the significance of daily accomplishments, no matter how minor they appear. When you return to your diary, you're rewarded with a gallery of these modest victories, which collectively remind you that every step you take, no matter how small, matters.

Reflecting on Challenges:

The road to greater flexibility and mobility is not always an easy one. It frequently entails overcoming obstacles and dealing with setbacks. Your journal becomes a refuge, a safe haven where you can work through these difficulties. When difficulties arise, and progress becomes unattainable, your notebook is a confidant, a place where you may openly share your thoughts and emotions.

You can transform problems into chances for progress in your diary. Whether it's the frustration of a plateau or the worry of a seemingly impossible challenge, expressing your feelings may be incredibly cathartic. It's a discharge of the emotional baggage that numerous challenges bring. You begin the path to knowledge and resolution by acknowledging and embracing these emotions in your notebook.

Reflective writing allows you to gain perspective on the difficulties you face. You can investigate the underlying causes of these difficulties, potentially uncovering patterns or triggers. This understanding might be vital in developing solutions and strategies to address future difficulties. As a result, your notebook becomes a tool for self-discovery and problem-solving, making it a useful companion on your path to greater flexibility and mobility.

A Source of Motivation:

Your journal, a repository of your journey's memories, is a never-ending source of inspiration. As you read through the pages, you're reminded of your progress and how far you've come, retracing your steps. It's like a visual timeline of your triumphs, a monument to your dedication. The act of revisiting previous entries rekindles your determination, propelling your enthusiasm for the voyage ahead.

The visual representation of your accomplishments in your journal instills a powerful sense of pride and empowerment. You see concrete evidence of your dedication, not just words and sketches. This validation boosts your drive by reminding you that you're on a road of progress and self-improvement. Your journal becomes a dynamic source of inspiration, a daily reminder that you can attain the goals you've set for yourself.

Holding Yourself Accountable:

Inscribing your aims and intentions in your journal is like making an ink commitment. This written contract reflects your hopes and dreams, transforming them into concrete pledges. It's a promise to oneself, a commitment that goes beyond just thoughts and aspirations.

This written commitment is a strong motivator. Your commitment to stick to your flexibility and mobility goals carries a weight that keeps you focused and determined. Your journal becomes a symbol of your dedication, a reminder of your dedication to your personal well-being, which serves as a driving force in your journey.

Identifying Patterns:

Your journal has a wealth of knowledge, a treasure trove of insights just waiting to be discovered. It is an effective tool for identifying patterns in your flexibility and mobility journey. As you review your entries, you may notice patterns relating to specific exercises, routines, or lifestyle aspects that influence your success. These patterns serve as guideposts, providing useful information about what works best for you.

Identifying these patterns has the potential to be revolutionary. It allows you to optimize the efficacy of your efforts by fine-tuning your routines. Perhaps you've seen that certain stretches provide more substantial effects, or that certain behaviors or environmental factors have a favorable or bad impact on your flexibility. This knowledge enables you to customize your approach to meet your specific requirements. As a result, your diary serves as a compass, guiding you through your path more quickly and with a better awareness of what contributes to your growth.

Setting Goals:

Apart from documenting your journey, your journal is the perfect place to set, evaluate, and adapt your goals. Whether you're striving to increase your range of motion, reduce muscle stiffness, or enhance your overall well-being, your journal offers a structured platform to outline your objectives and track your progress toward achieving them.

Expressing Emotions:

Your journal offers a judgment-free zone where you can freely express your emotions, whether they stem from the exhilaration of a breakthrough or the frustration of a plateau. By acknowledging and processing your feelings, you can maintain a healthy perspective on your journey.

Evaluating Progress and Making Necessary Adjustments

The importance of continual review and adaptation in increasing flexibility and mobility cannot be overstated. It is critical to remember that growth and transformation are not linear processes when you begin to document your progress. Instead, they are frequently denoted by curves, bends, and, occasionally, forks in the road. Your notebook becomes your guide, allowing you to critically examine your course and make the necessary adjustments to keep you on track.

The Art of Self-Reflection:

One of the journal's key responsibilities is to act as a mirror, reflecting your progress on your journey back to you. It becomes a place for self-reflection, prompting you to step back and assess your path. This part of self-reflection is critical because it allows you to obtain a clear perspective on the trajectory of your trip.

Begin by returning to previous entries on a regular basis. You'll discover that your journal is more than simply a collection of words and figures as you read through it. It's a patchwork of your memories, emotions, and life events. When you review your entries, you start on a journey through your own history, rekindling recollections of both major and minor accomplishments. You can see how far you've progressed and how your adventure has changed over time. In this sense, your diary functions as a personal time machine, allowing you to travel back in time to revisit your old self and celebrate your growth and triumphs.

Understanding Progress:

Flexibility and mobility progress frequently unfold in complicated and nuanced ways. It's not simply about being able to touch your toes or stretch your arms a little further. Progress also means feeling more at ease in your body, having fewer aches and pains, and having more freedom in your daily life. Your journal is a tool for recognizing and celebrating these intangible growth qualities.

Consider adding qualitative aspects to your journal to understand your development better. Along with documenting bodily changes or accomplishments, write down how you feel after a session. Is there a feeling of lightness, relaxation, or better vitality? How does your increased flexibility affect your daily life? These qualitative indicators are equally useful in assessing your progress. You acquire a more holistic view of your growth if you analyze both your trip's quantitative and qualitative parts.

Recognizing Plateaus:

Plateaus are regular occurrences on any journey, whether it is in physical fitness or in life in general. They are the periods of time when progress appears to slow or stall. Understanding and accepting that plateaus are a normal part of the process is critical. They do not indicate regression but rather an opportunity to experiment with and improve your technique.

Your journal is crucial in identifying and working through plateaus. Reviewing previous entries, you may find trends connected with periods of slower growth. Perhaps certain routines or workouts appear to be less successful during certain phases. Recognizing these trends allows you to change your routines proactively, experimenting with new exercises or strategies to break through plateaus.

In this way, your diary transitions from a passive record to an active instrument for adaptation, assisting you in navigating these difficult stages with strength and grace.

Setting Realistic Expectations:

Keeping your expectations realistic and adaptable is critical as you assess your progress. Progress does not necessarily happen in a straight line. There may be days when your flexibility appears to regress significantly, or you face impediments that briefly impede your progress. Your journal can be a gentle reminder that these feelings are natural and do not undermine the value of your entire trip.

Embrace the concept of non-linearity as part of your growth in your journal. If you have setbacks or delayed development, keep a journal to convey your emotions and thoughts. This reflective approach allows you to accept the facts of the journey and, if necessary, change your expectations. Remember that your journey to greater flexibility and mobility is a marathon, not a race. Slower, more contemplative segments are just as necessary as fast-paced segments. Your journal assists you in maintaining a balanced perspective by emphasizing the value of perseverance and patience as you work toward your goals.

Adapting and Refining Your Routine:

Your journal also catalyzes change and improvement. Reflecting on your journey, you may notice that certain routine components require modification. This could be related to the types of workouts you're doing, the length of your sessions, or the frequency with which you undertake them. You can use your journal as a blank canvas to brainstorm and document potential improvements.

When you identify areas needing adjustment, view them as opportunities to improve your routine. Experiment with new exercises, approaches, or durations and record the results. As a result, your journal becomes a dynamic workspace where you may create and implement personalized techniques to maximize your journey.

Seeking Guidance:

Your journal might be a chat with yourself or a mentor, as well as a private monologue. Seek advice from professionals or more experienced people in flexibility and mobility. Keep a log of these interactions. External perspectives can be essential for strengthening your trip, whether it's guidance from a physical therapist, insights from a yoga instructor, or wisdom from a seasoned athlete.

Working with professionals or subject matter experts helps you to benefit from their knowledge and experience. These insights can motivate you to change and adapt your daily routine. Your journal serves as a reservoir for this collective wisdom, allowing you to recollect and apply these lessons as you progress.

Tracking Health and Well-being:

Your general health and well-being are important considerations in your quest for increased flexibility and mobility. It's critical to realize that your journey isn't just about physical changes. It also includes your mental and emotional health. Your journal can help you keep track of various aspects of your life.

Consider writing about your mental and emotional experiences in your journal. Track how your flexibility and mobility practices affect your mood, stress levels, and overall mental wellness. Do you have less stress, better sleep, or more mental clarity? These qualitative indicators of well-being are critical components of your journey. You'll better grasp how your efforts affect all elements of your life if you acknowledge them in your notebook.

Taking Note of Lifestyle Factors:

Aside from your flexibility and mobility routines, lifestyle factors have a big impact on your success. Your journal can serve as a repository for these outside effects. Keep track of your everyday behaviors, such as sleep patterns, eating, and hydration. These aspects of your lifestyle are connected with your path of flexibility and mobility.

As you assess your development, note how lifestyle factors affect your flexibility and mobility. Do your dietary choices have an impact on your energy levels during practice? Does your sleeping pattern affect your overall physical performance? These observations can help you make the required lifestyle changes to enhance your journey further.

Planning for the Future:

Your journal is a tool for planning the future as well as a reflection of the past and present. Consider setting new goals and objectives as you assess your progress. Outline the steps needed to achieve these objectives in your journal.

Your journal can serve as a compass, pointing you in the right direction. Setting fresh goals makes your trip interesting and dynamic. You're more likely to stay motivated and devoted to your flexibility and mobility routines if you chronicle your goals.

In summary, assessing your progress and making appropriate adjustments is an essential part of your flexibility and mobility journey. Your journal is really important in this process. It is both a mirror and a compass, guiding you through plateaus and setbacks on your trip. Setting reasonable expectations, embracing non-linear development, adapting and refining routines, seeking help, and tracking your general well-being and lifestyle factors are all possible with a notebook. Finally, your journal serves as a dynamic area for growth and transformation, allowing you to navigate the challenges and possibilities that come along the way.

Setting Achievable Goals to Maintain Motivation

Setting achievable goals is a cornerstone of maintaining motivation and momentum in your flexibility and mobility journey. These goals provide a sense of direction and purpose, offering a clear path for your efforts. In your journal, you'll discover that goal-setting is not just about where you want to go but how you'll get there.

The Significance of Setting Goals:

Imagine a ship sailing without a destination. It might move but will do so aimlessly, without a purpose or direction. Similarly, setting goals is like charting your course in your journey to enhance flexibility and mobility. These goals become your North Star, guiding you toward a specific destination. They give your efforts purpose and provide a means to measure your progress.

When you set achievable goals, you create a framework for your journey. These goals serve as motivation and offer a tangible endpoint for your efforts. This process in your journal is a testament to your dedication and focus. It's an intentional exercise that shapes your daily routines and provides a sense of fulfillment and accomplishment.

Types of Goals:

In your flexibility and mobility journey, it's essential to recognize that not all goals are created equal. Goals can vary in scope, time frame, and specificity. In your journal, you can delineate different types of goals that serve various purposes.

- **Short-term Goals:** These are objectives that you aim to achieve within a relatively brief time frame. They are like steppingstones, marking your progress along the way. Short-term goals can be as simple as increasing your daily stretching duration or mastering a specific yoga pose.

- **Long-term Goals:** These are your larger aspirations, the ultimate destinations you want to reach in your journey. Long-term goals can be more ambitious, such as achieving a full split or being able to perform a challenging advanced stretch. These goals may take months or even years to accomplish.

- **Process Goals:** These goals are centered on the journey rather than the destination. They focus on the daily routines and practices that lead to progress. Process goals might involve committing to several stretching sessions per week or consistently practicing mindfulness during your routine.

- **Outcome Goals:** Outcome goals are the end results you're striving for, such as achieving a specific level of flexibility or mobility. In your journal, you can outline the steps and actions needed to reach these outcomes.

- **Performance Goals:** Performance goals are about improving your abilities and skills. For example, your goal might be to increase your range of motion in a particular stretch by a certain percentage.

- **Maintenance Goals:** Once you've achieved a particular level of flexibility or mobility, maintenance goals become relevant. These goals focus on sustaining your progress and preventing regression. You can use your journal to outline routines that help you maintain your current level of flexibility and mobility.

- **Adjustment Goals:** In your journey, you may encounter setbacks or plateaus. Adjustment goals come into play when you need to adapt your routines or strategies to overcome these challenges. Your journal serves as a space for brainstorming and recording these adjustment goals.

SMART Goals:

Effective goal-setting follows a specific framework, often referred to as SMART goals. This acronym stands for Specific, Measurable, Achievable, Relevant, and Time-bound. Applying the SMART criteria to your goals in your journal can enhance their effectiveness.

- **Specific:** When setting goals, it's essential to be specific about what you want to achieve. Instead of a vague goal like "improve flexibility," a specific goal might be "increase hamstring flexibility to be able to touch toes comfortably."

- **Measurable:** Your goals should be quantifiable. You should be able to measure your progress and determine when you've achieved the goal. For instance, you can measure your hamstring flexibility by recording how close you are to touching your toes.

- **Achievable:** Goals should be realistic and attainable. You can use this criterion in your journal to assess whether your goals align with your current abilities and resources.

- **Relevant:** Goals should be relevant to your journey and your overarching objectives. They should connect to your pursuit of enhanced flexibility and mobility.

- **Time-bound:** Each goal should have a specific time frame for completion. For example, you might set a goal to achieve a specific range of motion within three months. This time frame creates a sense of urgency and helps you stay focused.

Setting Goals in Your Journal:

Your journal is the perfect place to record and refine your goals. When setting goals, consider your current abilities, preferences, and any specific challenges you face. In your journal, outline your goals, specifying their type (short-term, long-term, etc.), and apply the SMART criteria.

Consider these tips when setting goals in your journal:

- **Start with short-term goals**: Begin with achievable, short-term goals. These goals provide quick wins and motivate you as you work towards larger, long-term aspirations.

- **Make your goals personal:** Your goals should resonate with your personal motivations and desires. In your journal, express why each goal is meaningful to you.

- **Create a sense of progression:** Your goals can build upon each other. As you achieve one goal, set a new one that pushes you further. This sense of progression enhances your journey's dynamic nature.

- **Periodically review and adjust goals:** Goals aren't set in stone. As you evaluate your progress, be open to adjusting your goals. Your journal can be a space for documenting any goal adjustments to stay aligned with your evolving abilities and aspirations.

- **Use visualization:** Visualize yourself achieving your goals. Your journal is a place for creative expression, and you can incorporate visual elements, such as drawings or vision boards, to help manifest your goals.

In Summary: Setting achievable goals is a powerful motivator in your flexibility and mobility journey. Your journal serves as a space for articulating these goals, making them tangible, and refining them to align with the SMART criteria. Goals provide a sense of purpose and direction, guiding your daily efforts. They come in various forms, from short-term achievements to long-term aspirations, and you can use your journal to map out your entire goal-setting journey. Ultimately, your journal becomes a testament to your dedication and intention, offering a path toward fulfilling your flexibility and mobility goals.

Chapter 11

Additional Resources and

Further Learning

As you progress in your senior years toward improved flexibility and mobility, you'll discover many resources and opportunities to support and enhance your efforts. This chapter delves into these resources and opportunities for additional learning, which range from books and online videos to fitness classes and local workout groups.

Recommending Books, Online Videos, and Resources for Senior Flexibility and Mobility

In this day and age of digital connectivity, there is a wealth of information available to help you better comprehend senior flexibility and mobility. Books, online videos, and digital resources are valuable resources for anyone wishing to improve their mobility and flexibility in their golden years.

The World of Books:

Books have traditionally been considered portals to a wide realm of information and inspiration. Books are a timeless and dependable resource for seniors who want to improve their flexibility and mobility. The benefit of turning to the printed word is the depth and breadth of coverage that books provide on the subject. They are dependable friends, guiding seniors through the complexities of exercises, stretching techniques, and the science of flexibility.

Exploring the world of books may provide seniors with expert advice and helpful insights. Numerous books have been written by authors and experts in the domains of fitness, physical therapy, and wellness that cater exclusively to the requirements of older persons. These authors frequently draw on years of experience, study, and a deep grasp of seniors' specific challenges and objectives. Their words educate and motivate, providing a sense of purpose and desire for greater flexibility and mobility.

The everlasting accessibility of books distinguishes them as an irreplaceable resource. Seniors can read and re-read at their own pace, allowing the information to sink in gradually and become ingrained in their fitness path. The world of books is a treasure trove of insight and encouragement, whether it's a guidebook on easy stretching, an in-depth manual on enhancing joint health, or an inspirational memoir of a senior's transformation via fitness.

Books to Consider:

1. **Stretching for Seniors: A Step-by-Step Guide to Doing Safe Stretches by Sue Hitzmann**: This book offers an array of stretches specifically designed for seniors, emphasizing safety and effectiveness.

2. **Yoga for Seniors:** Simple Stretches for Whole-Body Flexibility by Michelle Pitt: Yoga is renowned for enhancing flexibility and balance, and this book focuses on gentle poses tailored for seniors.

3. **The Miracle Ball Method for Seniors**: Easy, Gentle Exercises by Elaine Petrone: Elaine Petrone's approach combines self-massage and stretching using small balls, offering an accessible way to improve flexibility and mobility.

4. **Younger Next Year for Women: Live Strong, Fit, and Sexy — Until You're 80 and Beyond by Chris Crowley and Henry S. Lodge**: Although not exclusively for seniors, this book provides a comprehensive guide to maintaining fitness and mobility as you age.

5. **The Anatomy of Stretching by Brad Walker:** Understanding the anatomy of your muscles and how they work can be invaluable for seniors looking to improve flexibility.

Navigating the Digital Landscape:

Those who prefer a more visual or interactive approach to learning will find a wealth of materials in the digital sphere. For seniors seeking immediate support and visual illustrations, online channels, particularly YouTube, have become havens. A large community of fitness instructors, yoga specialists, and physical therapists generously share their knowledge on all things connected to flexibility and mobility.

The beauty of online videos is their accessibility and variety. Seniors can explore many exercises, stretching routines, and mobility-enhancing procedures with only a few mouse clicks. These videos cater to a wide range of fitness levels and interests, from mild stretching for beginners to advanced yoga routines. The guidance is not only informative but also entertaining, as teachers guide you through the motions with clarity and encouragement. Whether you want to improve your range of motion, reduce joint stiffness, or simply keep active, the digital environment brings you a world of opportunities for seniors who want to improve their flexibility and mobility.

Online Videos and Channels to Explore:

1. **Eldergym (YouTube Channel):** Eldergym offers a variety of videos focused on senior fitness, including gentle stretching and mobility exercises.

2. **HASfit (Heart and Soul Fitness, YouTube Channel):** HASfit provides a broad range of workouts tailored for different fitness levels, including seniors. Their senior workouts emphasize safety and effectiveness.

3. **Yoga With Adriene (YouTube Channel):** Adriene Mishler's yoga videos are suitable for all ages and offer a gentle yet effective approach to enhancing flexibility and balance.

4. **Physiotherapy UQ (YouTube Channel):** This channel, created by the University of Queensland, offers videos on improving flexibility and mobility, particularly for those dealing with common age-related issues.

5. **SilverSneakers (Official Website):** SilverSneakers is a program specifically designed for older adults, and they offer online workout videos as part of their services.

Digital Resources and Websites:

The internet has become a vital gateway to a world of information and support for seniors wishing to improve their flexibility and mobility in the modern day. Aside from traditional books and films, a plethora of websites and digital resources are specifically designed to meet the specialized needs of older individuals.

These digital platforms function as virtual libraries, providing many materials such as enlightening articles, research findings, and practical stretches.

One of the primary benefits of these digital tools is their current information. Seniors can access the most recent studies and advice on flexibility and mobility. Many websites offer step-by-step guidance, ensuring that older folks can stretch safely and effectively. Whether you're interested in the science of flexibility or looking for precise instructions on specific exercises, the digital environment is a useful resource for seniors on their path to better health.

Websites to Explore:

1. **The National Institute on Aging (NIA):** The NIA offers a wealth of resources on healthy aging, including articles on exercise and stretching for seniors.

2. **Harvard Health Publishing:** Harvard Health Publishing provides articles on fitness and mobility, including tips for staying active as you age.

3. **American Council on Exercise (ACE):** ACE offers a range of fitness articles, including those focused on senior fitness and flexibility.

4. **Senior Exercise Central:** This website is dedicated to senior fitness and provides various resources, including articles and exercise guidelines.

5. **StretchCoach.com:** StretchCoach.com, founded by Brad Walker, offers various stretching resources and articles.

When exploring books, online videos, and digital resources, consider the following:

- **Diversify Your Sources:** Don't rely solely on one book or website. Explore a variety of sources to gain diverse perspectives and insights.

- **Check Credentials:** Ensure that the creators of these resources have relevant qualifications and expertise in the field of senior fitness and mobility.

- **Progress Gradually:** Not all exercises or routines may suit your current flexibility and mobility level. It's crucial to progress at a pace that aligns with your abilities and listen to your body's signals.

- **Combine Knowledge with Practice:** Knowledge is most effective when put into action. Don't just read or watch; apply what you learn to your daily routine.

As you go through these resources, you'll notice that they provide a comprehensive grasp of senior flexibility and mobility. Books provide in-depth knowledge, while online videos provide visual instruction and digital resources provide the latest findings and perspectives. As you use these excellent tools, your journey toward greater mobility and freedom grows deeper and more informed.

Encouraging Participation in Online Senior Fitness Classes

The internet is a hub for possibilities to engage with exercise and wellness programs developed specifically for elders in an increasingly digital world. Because of its accessibility and effectiveness in boosting mobility, strength, and overall well-being, online senior fitness sessions have grown in popularity. We'll look at virtual fitness classes and why they're a great alternative for seniors who want to improve their flexibility and mobility.

The Digital Fitness Landscape:

In recent years, the digital fitness landscape has undergone substantial change. Seniors now have access to a wide range of fitness programs from the comfort of their own homes thanks to the growth of high-speed internet and the introduction of video streaming platforms.

Why Seniors Should Consider Online Fitness Classes:

1. **Accessibility:** One of the primary advantages of online fitness classes is their accessibility. You can join a class from anywhere with an internet connection. This convenience is particularly beneficial for seniors who may have mobility issues or live in areas with limited access to in-person fitness facilities.

2. **Variety:** Online platforms offer an extensive variety of fitness classes. Whether you're interested in gentle stretching, yoga, low-impact aerobics, or strength training, you'll find a class that suits your preferences and needs. This variety allows you to explore different forms of exercise to enhance your flexibility and mobility.

3. **Expert Guidance:** Many online fitness classes are led by certified fitness instructors specializing in senior fitness.

These instructors have the expertise to design safe and effective workouts that cater to older adults' unique needs and challenges.

4. **Customized Workouts:** Online senior fitness classes often provide options for different fitness levels. This means that whether you're a beginner or have some prior experience, you can choose a class that aligns with your current fitness level. This customization is essential for a safe and enjoyable exercise experience.

5. **Community and Interaction:** Some online fitness platforms incorporate community features, allowing participants to interact with each other and with the instructor. This sense of community can boost motivation and make the experience more enjoyable.

Recommended Online Senior Fitness Classes:

1. **SilverSneakers:** SilverSneakers offers a range of online classes designed specifically for older adults. These classes include cardio, strength training, yoga, and more. If you have a SilverSneakers membership through your Medicare plan, these classes may be available to you for free.

2. **YMCA 360:** The YMCA offers YMCA 360, an online platform with a variety of workout videos, including options for seniors. They cover everything from chair exercises to yoga.

3. **AARP's Virtual Community Center:** AARP provides an online community center with fitness classes, workshops, and social events designed for seniors. The classes are free to access.

4. **Local Fitness Centers and Studios:** Many local fitness centers and yoga studios now offer virtual classes, so you can continue to engage with your favorite instructors or explore new classes from home.

Tips for Getting the Most Out of Online Fitness Classes:

- Choose a Suitable Space: Designate a comfortable and clutter-free area in your home for your workouts. Ensure good lighting and ventilation.

- Use Proper Equipment: Depending on the class, you may need some basic equipment like resistance bands, yoga mats, or small dumbbells. Having the right gear can enhance your experience.

- Set Realistic Goals: While online classes can be highly beneficial, it's essential to set realistic goals and pace yourself. Listen to your body, and don't push too hard, especially if you're just starting.

- Stay Consistent: Consistency is key to seeing progress in flexibility and mobility. Try to stick to a regular schedule for your online fitness classes.

- Hydrate and Fuel: Don't forget to stay hydrated and have a light snack before your class to keep your energy levels up.

Safety Considerations:

When taking online fitness classes, always put safety first. Before beginning a new fitness regimen, contact your healthcare physician if you have any pre-existing health ailments or concerns. Furthermore, make sure that the instructor in your selected class emphasizes safety and provides modifications for different fitness levels.

Online senior exercise programs have become a lifesaver for individuals wishing to enhance their flexibility and mobility. These sessions, with their accessibility, expert coaching, and variety, provide an excellent chance for seniors to embark on a fitness path that can lead to improved well-being and a higher quality of life.

Joining Local Senior Exercise Groups or Classes

While online fitness classes are a convenient choice, participating in local senior exercise groups or classes can provide a unique and enriching experience. These in-person gatherings provide social contact, personalized coaching, and the opportunity to connect with others in your neighborhood who share your interests. In this section, we'll look at the advantages of joining a local senior fitness group and how to choose the best one for you.

The Power of Community:

Humans are fundamentally social beings, and community is critical to our well-being, particularly as we age. Local senior fitness groups and programs provide opportunities for social interaction, which can improve your general health.

Benefits of Local Senior Exercise Groups:

1. **Social Interaction:** Loneliness and social isolation can adversely affect physical and mental health. Joining a local exercise group provides regular social interaction,

helping combat feelings of isolation and promoting a sense of belonging.

2. **Motivation and Accountability:** When you are part of a group, you're more likely to stay committed to your fitness routine. The sense of accountability to your fellow participants and the instructor can be a powerful motivator.

3. **Personalized Guidance:** In a local group setting, instructors can provide more personalized guidance, tailoring exercises to suit your specific needs and abilities. This level of attention is often challenging to achieve in online classes or solo workouts.

4. **Variety of Activities:** Local senior exercise groups often offer a variety of activities, from yoga and tai chi to strength training and dance. This diversity allows you to explore different forms of exercise and discover what you enjoy most.

5. **Mental Stimulation:** Interacting with others and learning new exercises can provide cognitive stimulation, essential for mental health. Engaging in group activities keeps your mind active and alert.

How to Find the Right Senior Exercise Group:

Finding the right local senior exercise group can be a rewarding endeavor. Here are some steps to guide you in your search:

1. **Ask Your Healthcare Provider:** Consult with your healthcare provider before joining any exercise group. They can offer insights into what types of activities are suitable for your current health and fitness level.

2. **Explore Local Community Centers:** Many community centers, YMCAs, and senior centers offer exercise classes for older adults. Visit their websites or give them a call to inquire about their offerings.

3. **Check Local Gyms and Studios:** Local gyms and fitness studios may provide senior-focused classes or group sessions. Explore options in your area and ask about trial classes or introductory sessions.

4. **Attend Senior Expos and Health Fairs:** Senior expos and health fairs often feature local organizations that cater to older adults. These events can be an excellent way to connect with different groups and gather information.

5. **Inquire About Class Schedules:** Consider your availability and preferences when choosing a group.

Some classes are held in the morning, while others may be in the afternoon or evening. Find a schedule that aligns with your routine.

6. **Visit a Class as an Observer:** Before committing, you can ask if it's possible to observe a class to understand the instructor's teaching style and group dynamics. This can help you determine if it's the right fit.

7. **Connect with the Instructor:** Building a rapport with the instructor is essential. Discuss your fitness goals and any specific limitations or concerns. A good instructor will be willing to accommodate your needs.

8. **Consider the Location:** Evaluate the location of the group. It should be easily accessible and, if possible, close to your home. Convenience is a crucial factor in maintaining consistency.

Safety Considerations:

Safety should be a top priority when joining a local senior exercise group. Here are some safety considerations to keep in mind:

- **Health Assessment:** Consult with your healthcare provider to ensure you're physically capable of participating in the chosen activities.

- **Instructor Qualifications:** Verify the qualifications and certifications of the instructor. They should have experience in leading exercises for older adults.

- **Proper Warm-up and Cool-down:** Ensure the class incorporates appropriate warm-up and cool-down routines to prevent injury.

- **Communication:** If you have any pre-existing medical conditions or limitations, communicate them to the instructor to ensure that exercises are adapted to your needs.

- **Hydration and Nutrition:** Stay hydrated and have a light snack before class to maintain energy levels.

Local senior fitness groups provide the ideal combination of physical activity, social interaction, and personalized supervision. They foster a sense of community, improving your general well-being and making your journey to greater flexibility and mobility more enjoyable. So, take the first step by joining a local group and viewing each workout session as an opportunity to connect, learn, and grow with people in your community.

Chapter 12

Conclusion and Encouragement

As we get to the end of this guide, consider your transforming journey to improve your flexibility and mobility. You've not only received valuable knowledge, but you've also made tangible efforts to improve your overall well-being. In this last chapter, we'll review the importance of flexibility and mobility for seniors, urge you to incorporate these exercises into your everyday routines, and celebrate your tremendous success and improved quality of life.

Recap of the Importance of Flexibility and Mobility for Seniors

As we come to the end of this guide, it's important to remember how important flexibility and mobility are in the lives of seniors. The journey you've taken, digging into the complexities of these facets of physical health, has shed light on their importance. Flexibility and mobility, particularly in older people, are more than just characteristics; they are the foundations of a vigorous and satisfying existence. In this conclusion, we will emphasize their significance by considering how they impact daily experiences and quality of life.

The aging process causes numerous changes in the body. The gradual loss of muscular mass and strength is one of the most noticeable changes. This natural condition, known as sarcopenia, normally begins around the age of 30 and accelerates around the age of 50. Muscle mass loss implies less muscle is available to support and move the body, decreasing strength and overall physical performance. This manifests in everyday challenges for elders, such as lugging groceries, climbing stairs, or getting in and out of chairs. The vitality of independence is inextricably associated with the ability to execute these routine tasks without assistance.

As we've discussed earlier, the loss of muscle mass and strength isn't an irreversible fate. With dedicated exercises, it's possible to counteract this decline, enhancing strength and resilience.

Connective tissue changes exacerbate the difficulty of maintaining flexibility and mobility in seniors. Tendons and ligaments, which are important structural components of the body, lose flexibility as we age. This decrease in flexibility makes maintaining a large range of motion more difficult. Joints may stiffen and become less flexible, restricting one's ability to move freely. Imagine attempting to bend down and tie your shoelaces only to discover that your body does not allow such a simple maneuver. In such cases, frustration and potential loss of independence are obvious.

Osteoarthritis, which is common among seniors, can cause joint pain and movement limits. This common ailment can be especially aggravating since it can inhibit physical exercise and promote a sedentary lifestyle, increasing joint stiffness. It's not just about being uncomfortable; it's about how physical constraints can diminish one's freedom and quality of life. The capacity to move freely and comfortably is critical for seniors to participate in daily activities such as walking and climbing stairs, as well as getting in and out of chairs. Mobility is the essence of freedom, and it is related to a positive self-image and a lower chance of falling.

The topic of falls leads us to another critical component of elder health. A loss of balance and coordination frequently accompanies aging. Standing on one leg or walking on uneven terrain can become difficult and potentially dangerous. Reduced balance can also increase the probability of falls and the injuries that may result. Many elders are concerned about the potential implications of a fall, such as fractures and lengthy healing periods. Maintaining and strengthening balance is thus an issue of physical and emotional wellness.

Chronic health issues are usually companions in later life. Conditions such as osteoporosis and diabetes, which can alter bone density, circulation, and overall physical function, affect flexibility and mobility. Osteoporosis causes a decrease in bone density, making bones more prone to fractures. Diabetes, on the other hand, impairs circulation and nerve function, potentially leading to problems with extremity sensation. These conditions create additional obstacles to maintaining or improving flexibility and mobility. They pose challenges, but they are not insurmountable. Seniors can manage these issues by working with healthcare specialists and incorporating flexibility and mobility exercises into everyday routines.

When considering the relevance of flexibility and mobility for seniors, it is evident that these abilities are more than just physical. They are intrinsically tied to sustaining independence and quality of life. You've learned about the aging process and how it affects your physical capabilities as you read through this guide. More significantly, you've learned practical exercises and ways to prevent these consequences, putting you on the road to increased independence, better balance, and a higher quality of life. Flexibility and mobility are not goals to be attained and then abandoned. They are lifelong pursuits, and with each stretch and exercise, you take a step toward a future filled with vitality, strength, and the freedom to embrace life's many joys.

Encouragement to Integrate These Exercises into Daily Routines

As you conclude this guide, armed with knowledge and a renewed determination to improve your flexibility and mobility, it's critical to remember that the journey you've begun has no end point; it's a road that will last the rest of your life. Your devotion and persistence in learning and performing these exercises are wonderful, and it's time to move on to the next critical step: incorporating them into your everyday routines.

The exercises and techniques you've learned aren't just a to-do list item; they're tools for improving the overall quality of your life. Increased flexibility and mobility advantages are not limited to a specific age or time frame. They are long-term assets that can help you age gracefully while maintaining your independence.

Imagine beginning your day with some gentle stretching. As you reach and bend, you feel your body awaken, and the stress of a good night's rest gradually go. This creates a positive tone for the rest of your day, and the benefits continue as you go about your business. Simple chores like bending to tie your shoelaces, reaching for objects on high shelves, and getting in and out of your car become easier. Your independence is protected while the frustration of stiff joints and limited movement gradually gives way to a sense of empowerment.

Integrating these exercises into your daily life is about caring for your mental health as well as your physical health. You may notice an increase in your self-esteem and self-worth as you follow these habits. The ability to perform tasks on your own boosts your self-esteem and sense of accomplishment. It serves as a reminder that being older does not imply being helpless; rather, it is a time to appreciate your strength and resilience.

Exercises for flexibility and mobility are also an investment in fall prevention. Falls are a prevalent issue among the elderly, and the potential for damage from a fall is something that many seniors worry about. By incorporating these exercises into your regular routine, you will become more agile and prepared to respond to unexpected balance issues. The fear of falling eventually fades, and you gain better confidence in your actions.

Regular stretching and mobility exercises can help you manage chronic health conditions more efficiently, in addition to lowering your risk of falling. A commitment to physical activity can help control conditions like osteoporosis and diabetes. Regular weight-bearing workouts, for example, can help improve bone density and lower the risk of fractures in people with osteoporosis. Diabetes management, on the other hand, frequently entails regulating blood sugar levels and maintaining a healthy weight. Physical exercise contributes to both of these goals, providing a holistic approach to health management.

Furthermore, these exercises provide you with a key to a higher quality of life in addition to retaining your independence. The ability to move freely and comfortably is crucial for participating in everyday activities such as going about the neighborhood and climbing stairs, as well as enjoying outdoor adventures or simply playing with your grandchildren. Mobility allows you to explore your surroundings and interact with your community without requiring assistance.

So, consider these exercises to be crucial components of your daily routine, just as eating a decent meal and getting enough sleep are. Incorporate them in the mornings, afternoons, and evenings. Your dedication has been admirable thus far, and now is the moment to take the opportunity to improve your life in ways you could never have dreamed. These are not tasks but rather acts of self-care and empowerment. They are a testament to your commitment to your personal well-being and a gateway to a future filled with vitality, strength, and the freedom to enjoy life's many pleasures. Your path continues, and with each stretch, you move closer to a life filled with flexibility and mobility.

Celebrating the Progress and Improved Quality of Life Achieved Through Enhanced Flexibility and Mobility

It's time to ponder and celebrate as you near the finish of this complete guide to senior flexibility and mobility. You've decided to improve your quality of life by prioritizing and improving your flexibility and mobility. In this section, we'll discuss the significance of acknowledging and celebrating your accomplishments and their tremendous impact on your general well-being.

Throughout this book, you've learned about the numerous advantages of maintaining and improving flexibility and mobility. These advantages cover life's physical, emotional, and psychological aspects, and they are all interconnected. Incorporating stretching and mobility exercises into your everyday routine has opened the road for a healthier, more vibrant way of living.

Physical Transformations:

Let's start with the physical changes. By committing to these exercises, you've most likely noticed significant improvements in your strength and range of motion. Perhaps you can reach objects on higher shelves without thinking twice or easily bend to tie your shoelaces. These may appear as minor successes, but they represent considerable progress toward increasing your independence. Completing routine tasks without assistance is a significant accomplishment and an inspiring experience.

Furthermore, your balance and coordination are likely to have improved. Your newfound steadiness is a great asset that leads to a lower risk of falls and injuries. Falls are a major issue for seniors, and the fear of losing one's balance may be quite upsetting. Your dedication to these workouts has essentially established a safety net beneath you, lowering your danger of falling and the potential consequences that come with it.

Emotional and Psychological Well-being:

Beyond the physical advantages, consider the emotional and psychological advantages you've received from your journey to improve flexibility and mobility. Not only has your physical body changed, but so has your mental state. Your sense of accomplishment and independence has significantly impacted your self-esteem and self-image. You may experience renewed pride and confidence in your abilities. Aging can bring thoughts of fragility, but you've revived a sense of empowerment by exercising your independence.

The psychological benefit of not constantly worrying about falling or harming yourself is enormous. The fear of falling can become a constant, anxiety-inducing concern for many seniors. You've greatly lessened this fear by increasing your balance and coordination. As a result, your mental well-being is likely to have increased, and you may have a more positive outlook on life.

Quality of Life Enhancement:

One of the most striking results of your dedication to flexibility and mobility exercises is an improved overall quality of life. Your improved independence in moving and engaging in daily activities is a priceless gift.

You are not limited by bodily discomfort or the limitations of your body. Your quality of life has reached new heights, whether it's a leisurely walk in the park, a visit to friends and family, or engaging in hobbies you enjoy.

This improved quality of life also extends to your personal relationships. The ability to retain contact with family and friends is priceless. You can participate actively in family gatherings, visit loved ones, and engage in social activities. These encounters lead to a more happy and enjoyable retirement, and better mobility helps you take advantage of these opportunities fully.

As you celebrate your progress and improved quality of life due to increased flexibility and mobility, keep in mind that this journey is far from over. Your commitment to these exercises is a lifelong commitment to your well-being, not a short-term commitment. Every day is a new chance to continue on your path to greater vitality, strength, and independence. While your journey may have started as a way to better your physical health, it has evolved into a comprehensive endeavor that affects every aspect of your life. It's a path of self-empowerment, resilience, and the continual celebration of a life well-lived. Congratulations on taking such important steps toward a future of flexibility, mobility, and limitless possibilities.